THE
ONE MINUTE or̲ s̲o̲ HEALER

Also by Dana Ullman

Discovering Homeopathy: Medicine for the 21st Century

Everybody's Guide to Homeopathic Medicines
(with Stephen Cummings, M.D.)

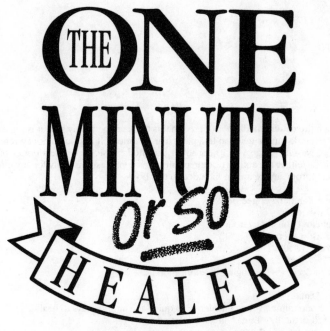

THE ONE MINUTE Or So HEALER

500 Quick and Simple Ways
to Heal Yourself Naturally

Dana Ullman, M.P.H.

Jeremy P. Tarcher/Perigee

Although the natural medicines offered in this book are generally safe, it is impossible to predict an individual's reaction to a particular treatment. If in doubt about a remedy or a reaction, we encourage you to consult a qualified physician or practitioner of natural medicine. Neither the author nor the publisher accepts responsibility for any effects that may occur from any treatment included in this book.

Jeremy P. Tarcher/Perigee Books
are published by
The Putnam Publishing Group
200 Madison Avenue
New York, NY 10016

Library of Congress Cataloging-in-Publication Data

Ullman, Dana.
    The one minute (or so) healer : 500 quick and simple ways to heal
  yourself naturally / Dana Ullman. — 1st ed.
        p.   cm.
      Includes index.
      ISBN 0-87477-667-8
      1. Homeopathy—Popular works.   I. Title.
    RX76.U46   1991   91-25743
    615.5'32—dc20   CIP

Jeremy P. Tarcher, Inc.
5858 Wilshire Blvd., Suite 200
Los Angeles, CA 90036

Design by Michele Lanci-Altomare
Illustrations by John Holmquist

Manufactured in the United States of America
10 9 8 7 6 5 4 3 2

Contents

▼

Contents

PART II. THE ONE-MINUTE (OR SO) HEALING STRATEGIES

PART III. RESOURCES

ACKNOWLEDGMENTS

▼

This book was written over a two-year period, but to gather the information required many lifetimes of experience of healers past and present.

There are innumerable friends and colleagues who provided input and inspiration to this book. A special thank you to Lynn Fraley, R.N., Dr. P.H.; James Gordon, M.D.; Ben Hole, M.D.; Sandra McLanahan, M.D.; Carolyn Reuben, C.A.; Michael Schmidt, D.C.; Jim Spira, Ph.D.; and Janet Zand Marcus, N.D., C.A. Richard Solomon, M.D. reviewed the entire manuscript for its medical accuracy, and his work is appreciated. A thank you to my friend Metece Riccio-Politi, who encouraged me to write this book when it was only in the idea stage, and to Steven Schmidt, who continually gives me inspiration.

I'd like to express appreciation to my assistants and co-workers, Robert Bruce Moody, Jocelyn Elder-Gray, Laura Elliot, and Sheila Halligan, who tell me when I'm funny *and* when I'm not.

My editor, Donna Zerner, deserves a very special thank you for her editing skills, her ideas, and her consistent and persistent vision of what this book could and should be. At times I had disturbing side effects from her surgical editing, but my words and I have survived to tell the story.

John Holmquist, this book's illustrator, put my cartoon concepts into visual form and I thank him for doing a superb job.

I am very lucky to have such a wonderful family and extended family who have been so supportive of me and my work. It's a pity that the powerful healing influence of having a loving family cannot be easily translated into a one-minute strategy.

A heartfelt thanks to my wife, Clare Ullman. Her ability to withstand my sense of humor at all hours of the day and night is truly herculean. Always giving feedback on my bedside personality, she has helped me refine my healing and loving abilities.

INTRODUCTION

······································▼·····································

THE DOCTOR IS IN

Becoming a healer in one minute is really no big deal. You've actually been working at healing longer than you think. Thousands of years of survival training have been built into your genes. From the moment of conception up to this very instant, every cell of your body has actively and continually defended itself against microbes, environmental assaults, and all types of stress. Perhaps most wonderful of all, your body has defended itself against you and the ravages you have inflicted on it. Occasionally, of course, you need some help. At times you may go to a health expert, and at other times, you learn a technique or two yourself.

This book will help you with the second option. It will increase your knowledge of what you can do to help the expert healer inside you do its work. Its premise is, if you take your disease lying down, you are apt to stay that way.

We commonly talk about the wisdom of the body, but all too often we don't think about the humor of the body. As magnificent as the human body is, it is a bit strange that our feet run and so does our nose, our mouth speaks and our stomach talks back, our knees knock and our ears ring. Hopefully, somebody is at home in there to respond to all this commotion.

When you think about it, the body is wonderfully creative in producing whatever symptoms it needs to get our attention. Aching, throbbing, cramping, itching, and inflaming are but some of the special effects it indulges in. It's also fond of sight gags and sound effects: it erupts, discharges, and discolors, and it emits gas and odors that get our attention (as well as those around us). It also calls attention to its problems by producing effects that make you feel feverish or fatigued, nauseous or nervous, and stiff or spastic. No bells and whistles, but just about everything else.

Even though there is a wisdom of the body, it isn't always easy to figure out its logic. What is the reasoning behind an allergy to cats? Some sort of survival mechanism developed to protect you from killer felines? Are the violent sneezing attacks nature's attempt to blow the life-threatening cats away? Every ailment has its mysteries.

This book will not try to answer all of your questions about health but it will answer many of them. It will also provide you with a deeper understanding of the innate healing powers within each person, give you some practical insights about the human body, and present you with sound and effective ways to heal it.

The first part of this book consists of twenty-two steps to healing, which outline the underlying principles of the healing process. These steps are worth your careful attention; healing is not simply a matter of applying a specific treatment to a specific problem, it is also about deepening your understanding of the human body and of nature, and an ability to use this knowledge to create a more healthy and joyful life. These steps help you see the bigger picture. They give you insight into why some healing techniques work and others don't, and why it's ultimately the way they are used that determines their effectiveness. But, while these ground rules for healing are basic and important, they are not the world's only healing principles. I hope each person will discover and use additional healing practices that work particularly well for them.

The second part of this book will give you the one-minute healing strategies, which are simple, effective treatments to help you help yourself. Besides being quick and easy, these methods are also safe—for the motto of any physician is "First, do no harm." Keep in mind, though, that they are not always one-minute cures. Rather, they are valuable strategies that will begin the healing process, for once healing is sparked, the inherent adaptive and self-healing capacities of the body take over.

Waking our inner doctor

The great physician and humanitarian Albert Schweitzer acknowledged the importance of every body's self-healing capacities when he said, "Each patient carries his own doctor inside him.

They come to us not knowing that truth. We are at our best when we give the doctor who resides within each patient a chance to go to work."

The primary purpose of this book is to make you aware of this inner doctor and to offer specific strategies that will let that doctor perform his (or her) daily miracles. Although there is much that physicians and other health professionals can do to prevent and treat disease, there is much more that each of us can do on our own. Your health is too important to leave it to someone else.

All healing is really self-healing. In the treatment of infection the drugs or herbs we take may have antibacterial properties, but unless your own immune system is strong enough, true healing does not take place. Surgery or a colonic may remove an unhealthy growth or substance, but unless your own defenses are strong enough to prevent it from coming back, real healing does not take place. Healthy foods and vitamin supplements may provide you with a nutritious diet when you're sick, but unless you have the internal building blocks to make use of these nutrients, healing does not take place.

To get healthy, your immune system must have a certain vigor and spark. Effective attitudes and treatments ultimately catalyze this spark so that the healing potential within awakens and spreads. Each step and strategy for healing in this book provides a little more understanding of your own body's processes; when applied, each does its part to increase and strengthen the body's self-healing capacities.

There will be times when you may not notice any immediate change after treating yourself with one of the strategies. Don't worry; there are enough strategies provided for each condition that one or more is likely to be helpful in some way. If you are not sure which strategy to use, you may need to tune in more to your own inner doctor (see step 4: "Seek Inner Wisdom"). If you're suffering in the meantime, you may need to get on better terms with your condition (see step 12: "Make Friends with Your Pain").

It is not the intent of this book to discourage the appropriate use of conventional medical treatment. Various modern medical diagnostic techniques can provide invaluable information about a person's state of health, and many modern medical treatments are literally lifesaving.

This book does, however, encourage caution in using certain drugs and medical procedures. While that doesn't mean that they should never be used, you are encouraged to think twice about using them. Try other, safer strategies first, or consult your health practitioner about the wisdom of their use for your particular problem.

The best way to heal yourself may be a collaborative approach which integrates conventional and alternative treatments (though there will be times you may want to rely just on one or the other). Whatever decision you make, a good place to begin is with step 1: "You Are the Most Important Member of Your Health-Care Team." You are the ultimate decision-maker—you're the one who's going to be stuck with your body, so if you don't take charge, who will?

It's been said that the best time for anyone to start the healing process is ten years ago. The second best time is today. If you're ready to start healing yourself *today*, this book will provide the strategies to help make it happen.

Part I

The Steps to Healing

1

······································▼······································

YOU ARE THE MOST IMPORTANT MEMBER
OF YOUR HEALTH-CARE TEAM

*The next major advance in the health of the American people
will be determined by what the individual
is willing to do for himself.*
John Knowles
Former President of the Rockefeller Foundation

According to the rules of the universe, you are not only required to play on your own health-care team, you are required to manage it, too.

To organize your health-care team you should first realize that doctors and other health-care professionals are your employees. That's right—the doctor doesn't pay you; you pay the doctor. The doctor is your expert consultant on medical matters. So, if this employee doesn't completely satisfy you in answering basic questions about your health, he should be replaced.

Bob Dylan once sang, "You don't need a weatherman to know which way the wind blows"; likewise, you don't always need a doctor to tell you how to feel better. Although professional medical care can be invaluable and sometimes crucial, there are many conditions that are more easily treated using simple home remedies, instead of complicated and expensive conventional medical treatment.

Western medicine offers what may be considered the Cadillac of medical care. But, just as it isn't always necessary, appropriate, or ecologically sound to drive a Cadillac, it isn't always necessary to receive Cadillac medical care. It makes more sense to treat yourself with home remedies for many common complaints. Such care will not only be cheaper and less risky, but will often be more effective. Simple home remedies can sometimes provide that extra nudge your body needs, while the big guns of medicine can be saved for more drastic situations.

What you do for yourself in the ways that you eat, exercise, deal with stress, and feel and express yourself can help prevent illness and promote health. This attention to your health doesn't have to be the chore that some people make it. A healthy lifestyle can be wonderfully invigorating, enlivening, and joyful, and if it isn't, you're doing something wrong.

Determining the healthiest things to do for yourself usually requires personal study, self-reflection, and expert assistance. Here's where organizing your own health team comes in.

People often put more energy into choosing an auto mechanic than they do into choosing their own doctor. To find a good doctor, it's necessary to do some homework. Ask your friends or other people you trust which doctors they recommend. Find out if the doctor is a good listener, explains things clearly, informs patients of various options available, encourages patient involvement in health, and is knowledgeable about self-care strategies.

In addition to seeking out conventional medical help, you should also consider adding to your team other assistants, perhaps an acupuncturist, homeopath, naturopath, chiropractor, psychologist, social worker, nutritionist, stress-management consultant, spiritual advisor, or exercise coach. This isn't to say that you need to consult all of these experts. As the manager of this team, you decide who to send in and when.

Whoever you choose, make certain that they do nothing *to* you, only *with* you. And if they don't directly discuss with you what you can do to improve your own health, they are not enlisting the help of the most important member of the health-care team.

Ultimately, even if your health practitioner gives you sound advice on what you can and should do to improve your health, you're the one who must fill this prescription. Good health advice is often ignored, and suing yourself for malpractice is not a viable option.

There is a tendency to blame the medical professional for not getting the patient better. Although this is sometimes true, it is important to remember that every time you point your finger at something else as the source of your problems, you also have three more fingers pointing back at you-know-who.

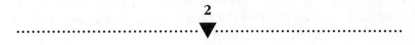

2

WHEN NATURE CALLS, ANSWER

We command nature only by obeying her.
Francis Bacon

One of the ways that your car tries to warn you of an impending problem is by flashing a light at you. A symptom of malfunction in your car is like a symptom of the body; it is trying to tell you something.

When your oil light comes on, do you try to unplug it? Probably not, and yet we commonly seek to turn off or suppress our symptoms as a way of dealing with them. However, like the car that has a flashing oil light, unless you do something to deal with the problem, it may get worse.

On the other hand, unlike warning signals in a car, the symptoms of the body do not simply represent a sign of something gone wrong. They are also adaptive responses of the body in its efforts to deal with stress or infection. By turning off this adaptive response, we inhibit our own ability to defend and heal ourselves.

A fever, for instance, is an important defense of the body. It is the way that the body creates an internally heated environment so that viruses and bacteria cannot survive as easily. During a fever, the body's white blood cells become more active, and the body's own antiviral chemical—interferon—is secreted in greater amounts. It is therefore not surprising that drugs that suppress fever can not only prevent the body from healing, but can also cause serious side effects.

Suppressing a symptom is like shooting the messenger because you don't like the message. The messenger may die, but the message remains the same.

A *symptom* is any phenomenon or circumstance accompanying an ailment and serving as evidence of it. So, when we treat a symptom, we are not necessarily healing the disease that is causing it; we are treating the phenomenon or circumstance of the illness, not the illness itself.

The common practice of treating a headache with painkillers is a classic example of this adversarial approach. Just the word *painkiller* lets you know that you are trying to destroy something. And yet, the head pain is only a symptom of the disease. Whether the headache results from the stress of a relationship or from overwork, a response to overeating, drinking too much coffee, or whatever, treating the head pain with a painkiller does nothing to address the source of the symptom. And to make things worse, the body now has to deal with a drug which is suppressing the body's effort to call attention to a problem.

We commonly mistake the symptoms themselves as the problem and we assume that we must rid ourselves of them. We then use various treatments that attempt to do just that. We try to eradicate the symptom, inhibit the disease, and think we're attacking the problem. What we are doing is trying to control, outwit, and dominate nature. In so doing, we are setting up an adversarial approach to dealing with our affliction.

The fighting language suggested by conventional drug treatment is the opposite of a mindset of working *with*, instead of against, the body's efforts. Instead of turning off symptoms, this gentler mindset is apt to favor approaches that attempt to strengthen the immune system, augment the person's own defenses, and nurture the body's own healing capacities.

Instead of ignoring our own symptoms or simply letting a doctor figure out what to do, we can use our illness as an opportunity to figure out what our symptoms are saying to us. They may be saying that something in us is out of balance with our environment, or that something in our environment is out of balance with us. Whatever method you choose to determine what this something is, illness is an opportunity to seek greater understanding of yourself and your interaction with the world. It is also an opportunity to begin to change yourself or your environment.

The human organism, however, has impressive—even incredible—adaptive healing capacities which have been developed and refined over millions of years. When we can learn to reestablish a healthy balance between our bodies and the world that surrounds us, the body is better able to work its wonders to heal itself.

We must listen carefully to our own symptoms, and we must listen carefully to what the world in which we live is saying to us. Robert Frost emphasized the importance of this listening when he wrote:

How many times it thundered before Franklin took the hint! How many apples fell on Newton's head before he took the hint! Nature is always hinting at us. It hints over and over again. And suddenly we take the hint.

Our bodies, too, give us hints all the time. Do you acknowledge these hints? Do you do something about them? Next time nature calls, answer.

3

........................▼........................

YOUR HEADBONE'S CONNECTED TO YOUR . . .

The human body is the best picture of the human soul.
Ludwig Wittgenstein

The mind and the body are undeniably interconnected. Anyone who doesn't recognize that the mind can readily create physical symptoms is cutting off the head at the neck. This "Marie Antoinette" style of medicine is a bit out of date.

Emotional and mental states have certain effects on the body; likewise, the body has the power to create certain emotional and mental states. You probably know of someone who became ill shortly after a crisis in the family, and you probably also know of someone who suffered from a lengthy or uncomfortable illness and became depressed, anxious, fearful, or a bit crazed as a result of it.

An integral aspect of Chinese medicine recognizes the connection between organ systems and emotional states. The liver, for instance, is related to anger, the lungs to depression, and the kidneys to fear. Thus, if a person has a diseased liver from drug or alcohol abuse, it is likely that they also experience (or are suppressing) more than a little anger. Likewise, a person with a lung condition usually breathes with difficulty, often leading them to feel more depressed than normal. Just as a depressed emotional state can lead to inhibited breathing, inhibited breathing can create a lethargic and depressed emotional state. It is no coincidence that the simple act of sighing, often due to the body's efforts to catch up on the oxygen deprivation resulting from inhibited breathing, is intertwined with feelings of sadness. The kidneys, which are situated just below the fight-or-flight adrenal glands, are directly affected by and directly affect the emotion of fear. Chinese medicine readily acknowledges the dynamic interplay between psyche and soma, for it recognizes that emotional disturbances are as likely to create physical disorders as physical disturbances are likely to create emotional disorders.

It is sometimes useful to know which came first—the psychological problem or the physical problem. However, this knowledge is not always obvious, and it isn't always helpful. It is of no value to try to extinguish the original match that started a forest fire—a fireman must put out the entire blaze, not just the initial flames. Likewise, the best strategy to deal with a sick person may be to treat the whole person. Although the phrase "treating the whole person" has recently become almost trite, it is nevertheless worthwhile to use various strategies concurrently, each of which attempts to heal one or more of the "blazes" in the body and in the mind. Treating liver problems, for instance, may require reducing drug and alcohol intake and reducing exposure to toxic substances, as well as increasing intake of vitamin A and green leafy vegetables, starting a relaxation program, and learning to express anger constructively. The second part of this book gives you helpful strategies that deal with specific problems from both a mind and a body perspective.

Using many healing methods at once is sometimes the best strategy, though another approach is to use a single method that focuses squarely on the primary source of the problem. If a person experiencing indigestion discovers that he is allergic to certain foods, it makes sense to avoid these foods rather than trying to get rid of the symptoms of the problem in other more indirect ways. Applying a specific treatment alone to what may be the primary irritation may create calm and promote effective healing.

Making the decision to try one approach or another to heal your mind and body problem should not be only a rational decision but also an intuitive one. Ask your right brain to help too. And while you're at it, you might also consider asking your headbone, your neckbone, your shoulderbone . . .

It's all connected.

4

SEEK INNER WISDOM

Direct your eye inward and you'll find a thousand regions in your mind yet undiscovered.
Henry David Thoreau

Psychologist Lawrence LeShan once remarked, "If the brain were so simple that we could understand it, we would be so simple that we couldn't."

Some brain researchers do not think of the brain as an *organ* of perception but as a *filter* of perception. The brain, they say, absorbs much more than we realize. They crudely estimate that we become aware of only about ten to fifteen percent of what the brain absorbs. The rest of the information becomes a part of our subconscious mind.

This may sound exciting, but what can you do with it? How can you get access to that other 85 to 90 percent?

One trick to getting access to the hidden wisdom of the brain is to not try. This Zen paradox has frequently been described by researchers. There are innumerable stories of scientists who were working on a specific problem for days, weeks, months, or years . . . and then, in a moment of relaxation, sometimes during sleep, a sudden insight came to them, providing the key piece of the puzzle.

Another trick to draw on subconscious information is to relax, meditate, and simply but directly ask a question that you want answered. Don't try to answer it yourself; simply listen and see if an answer comes to you. This process, at worst, gives you an opportunity to be clear on the question you want answered, and at best, it may help you tap into the deeper reaches of the brain and gain access to the information you need.

This exercise may also be used for healing. You can tune into your inner doctor and ask for a diagnosis or for advice on what you should do about your condition. This inner doctor may take the form of a person, an animal, or even an object. The information may come in the form of symbolic words, images, or gestures which have a special meaning. It may be a challenge to figure out what is being said, and yet, when considering the different possible meanings, people often notice that one interpretation feels right.

The inner doctor's suggestion for treatment may be something you can do for yourself, or it may be to seek professional treatment. Your inner doctor may not always recommend natural therapies; you may be encouraged to see a physician or even a surgeon. Your inner doctor may also suggest that the symptoms *are* the cure and that the best thing you can do is let the symptoms run their cycle without impediment.

Being a hard worker, your inner doctor also operates while you sleep; dreams are one of his mediums of communication. Like other processes that open up your subconscious mind, these messages are usually symbolic and require intuition to interpret. In order to prepare yourself for your doctor's advice, try repeating to yourself just before falling asleep, "I ask for guidance, and I allow the information I need to enter my dreams."

Get in touch with your inner wisdom; you are smarter than you think.

Of course, after you've gotten comfortable contacting your inner doctor, you can start tuning into your inner financial consultant if you're having money problems. You can tune into your inner coach if you want to improve your sports performance.

5

▼

TAKE RESPONSIBILITY FOR YOUR HEALTH, BUT DON'T TAKE BLAME FOR YOUR DISEASE

There are responsible persons, but there are no guilty ones.
Albert Camus

When people say that you are responsible for your health and to blame for your disease, they are exhibiting a classic case of *wellness-macho*. This machisimo attitude assumes that you have much greater power and influence over your health than you may actually have.

The assumption behind this belief is that we create our own reality. We are responsible for whatever infections we have because we have allowed ourselves to be infected. We are responsible for our chronic diseases because we have not done whatever was necessary to strengthen our own immune system. We are responsible for genetic diseases because our soul picked our own parents before we were born.

The extreme version of this attitude is that people allow drunk drivers to hit them, passengers knowingly choose to go on a plane that crashes, and the families in Love Canal were responsible for their exposure to environmental toxins. This attitude is not limited to New Age fanatics. Even during the Great Depression a large percentage of men blamed themselves for being out of work.

We do indeed cause various problems for ourselves, many more than most of us recognize. However, to think that we create everything that happens to us is to ignore the obvious and far-ranging influence of our physical and social environment. To assume that each individual creates his own fate is to have an incredibly egotistical view of the world.

One serious side effect of wellness-macho is the feeling of guilt it creates, and the last thing that a sick person needs is this additional emotional weight. To make matters worse, these guilt-ridden people then expend great energy searching for what they did to cause their misfortune, when their energy could be used more effectively if applied to healing.

Whether the notion that we create our own diseases seems perfectly logical or completely preposterous, one value that it does have is that it can help to empower the individual. It reminds us that we have the power to greatly influence our own lives. It encourages us to no longer blame others for our problems. We can find lessons to be learned in everything that happens to us. For instance, if you have weak knees, perhaps you may take this as a sign to stand up for yourself. If you have poor digestion, you simply have to be more conscious of eating healthy foods. If you have a headache, you may realize that you have to relax more often. On a more serious level, if you are paralyzed, you may need to learn how to ask for help from others. There is something valuable in the assumption that trying to learn from your circumstances is a much more effective strategy than being devastated by them.

Perhaps the best strategy to deal with wellness-macho is to recognize the difference between being responsible for your own health and being to blame for your illness. Reverend Jesse Jackson shed light on this when he told a high school audience, "You may or may not be responsible for being down, but you are responsible for getting up." Likewise, you may or may not be responsible for being ill, but you are responsible for doing something about it.

6

▼

THE TEN STEPS TO HEALTHY EATING

To eat is human, to digest divine.
Mark Twain

Even according to the American government, our Standard American Diet is SAD. If "you are what you eat" is true, many Americans may be more or less composed of Twinkies, Frosted Flakes, and Ding-Dongs. When you consider that the nutrients we ingest today become tomorrow's muscle, nerve, and brain cells, it is frightening to consider what becomes of a person who maintains a steady diet of junk food. It is no wonder that some people have Twinkie muscles, frosted nerves, and Ding-Dong brains.

Hippocrates, the father of western medicine, said, "Let food be your medicine." This doesn't necessarily mean that food is the only medicine, but it does emphasize that many foods have healing properties. Bananas, for instance, can help heal ulcers, onions can relieve bronchial congestion, mushrooms can inactivate certain viruses, and cranberry juice can cure urinary tract infections.

Although foods have the power to heal, they also have the power to cause harm. Milk products, wheat, eggs, and chocolate, for example, are common foods to which many people are allergic. Such foods may not only create digestive problems, but could also cause various symptoms including fatigue, recurrent headaches, and disturbing emotional and mental problems. As the old saying goes, One man's meat is another man's poison.

Finding the foods and combination of foods that are right for you is not always easy. Perhaps this is why one nutritionist in San Francisco calls herself an "interior decorator." Although there is little upon which all nutritionists agree, there are some generally recognized steps to healthy eating that—if you follow—will definitely prove beneficial.

14

There is no ideal nutrition program
for everyone

Not only do you have your own individual nutritional needs, these needs can change from season to season and year to year. Where and how you live also influences your nutritional needs. For example, people in cold climates need more caloric intake and need to eat more cooked foods than people in warm climates. The degree of physical activity or emotional stress in your life will affect your nutritional needs. Genetics also plays a role in determining your nutritional requirements because the body becomes accustomed to what its ancestors ate.

The type of food you eat is more important
than what vitamins and supplements you take

Many foods not only contain many common nutrients but also numerous trace elements that are important, even essential, for health. Chromium, boron, molybdenum, vanadium, and manganese are all important in maintaining health, and yet they are rarely included in the typical vitamin pill.

Foods also often have a complement of nutrients in them that make them easier to digest. Oranges, for instance, not only have vitamin C, they also have bioflavinoids, which help the body assimilate vitamin C more efficiently. Eating an orange, then, is a more efficient source of getting and assimilating important nutrients than popping a pill.

Eat fresh foods whenever possible

Food processing reduces the nutritional content of food. Frozen, canned and packaged foods will not be as nutritious as those that you make fresh.

Although our fast-paced modern lifestyle encourages a tendency to eat processed food, the time we save by consuming such fare we often lose suffering from its effects. Many fresh foods can be prepared easily and rapidly. The trick is learning how to make quick, natural, and fresh meals and snacks; there are numerous cookbooks now available that can help you to do this.

15

Eat low on the food chain

Pesticides accumulate in greater concentrations in animals, which are higher on the food chain than any other food. A vegetarian diet that consists primarily of whole grains, beans, vegetables, and fruits sharply reduces the level of exposure to pesticides and other toxins. Other benefits of a noncarnivorous diet are lower rates of heart disease, cancer, and numerous other acute and chronic illnesses. Talk to any vegetarian and you'll discover many more good reasons to avoid meat. A. Whitney Brown offers this one you probably *won't* hear: "I'm not a vegetarian because I love animals. I'm a vegetarian because I hate plants."

Eat organic foods whenever possible

Organic foods are not only free from exposure to toxic pesticides but also tend to have greater nutritional value because they are grown in soil made more fertile with organic fertilizers. Although it is still uncertain how much pesticide you can ingest without substantially disturbing bodily functions or causing illness, it is certainly a worthy goal to limit exposure to it.

When possible, it is worthwhile to find out if the foods you are buying come from the United States or another country. Many pesticides that are banned in this country are exported elsewhere and come back to this country in imported food. One more example of karma playing out its drama.

Organic foods are often more expensive than nonorganic foods, though this price difference will diminish as demand for these safer foods increases. In the meantime, the extra cost for organic foods is worth the peace of mind and health of body that they give.

The hunger reflex means that
you should eat

As simple as this sounds, many people eat whether they are hungry or not. Evolution has endowed our body with a sophisticated method of knowing when to eat. This hunger reflex informs us of our idiosyncratic needs. Some people are very hungry in the morning, others are not. Some people more efficiently digest food when they eat frequent small meals and tend to get sleepy after a large lunch or dinner.

Knowing when to stop eating is as important as knowing when to start. Malnutrition is not simply a condition of not having enough to eat; it can also occur when a person has too much to eat. It may be strange to call some obese people "malnourished," but technically, it's true. It is most healthful to err by undereating rather than overeating. Recent research has suggested that animals that were slightly underfed lived considerably longer than those that were overfed.

Chew your food

Each stage of digestion is dependent upon the previous stage, and the first stage of digestion is proper chewing. During this stage you are not only breaking down food so that it can more easily slide down your throat, you are saturating the food with important salivary enzymes which begin the digestive process. Chewing carbohydrates is particularly important because salivary enzymes help to digest them. Too rapid swallowing of carbohydrates means that the pancreas is forced to bear the extra burden of digesting them, and considering most people's sugar-laden diet, the pancreas is already overworked.

Some nutrition zealots recommend chewing food until it is liquid in the mouth. Although this may be an occasional worthy goal, it is enough to actively chew every bite of food before swallowing.

Think about it; if you don't chew your food, who will?

You are not what you eat; you are what you assimilate

Because we do not assimilate all the nutrients from the food we eat, it may be more appropriate to say that we are what we assimilate.

Even the healthiest people do not absorb all the nutrients they ingest. People with digestive disturbances or with food allergies are even less able to fully absorb the food they eat. Although research on this subject is still relatively limited, it is known that certain nutrients make absorption of other nutrients more difficult, while others make it easier. For instance, numerous foods and drinks inhibit calcium absorption, including grains, spinach, chard, rhubarb, chocolate, peanuts, walnuts, soybeans, alcohol, and caffeine. Foods that aid calcium absorption include citrus fruits, apples, broccoli, carrots, cabbage, tomatoes, onions, cauliflower, and dark green leafy vegetables.

Be aware of your emotional state while eating

Various emotional states can inhibit digestive juices and stifle the digestive process. If you are having an argument during a meal, poor digestion is almost inevitable. If you think that the food you are eating isn't good for you, your anxiety about it may make it true. If you are eating while feeling depressed, expect your digestion to be depressed also; and to make things worse, this sloweddown digestion may lead to unwanted weight gain.

Because we season our food with feelings every time we eat, next time you're at the dinner table, don't ask anyone to pass the guilt, fear, anxiety, or anger. Such emotions can disturb digestion and do not combine well with *any* foods. It is healthier and wiser to bless the food, bless the people with whom you are eating, and bless yourself. This is a healthy combination that best helps the proper assimilation of food for the body, mind, and soul.

Eat foods that feel good to you and avoid foods that don't

Though not usually written about in conventional nutrition journals or discussed at nutrition conferences, your instincts will often lead you to the healthiest foods for you. If you observe your body closely, you will notice that some foods feel good to you even when you're just thinking about them, while others may feel draining.

You may also notice that some foods that normally taste bad will taste better when you are acutely ill. For instance, lemons tend to taste less sour and may even taste sweet when you have a cold or cough. This is but one more example of how nature provides us with hints on how to heal ourselves, and why it is worthwhile to follow your food and drink instincts during acute stages of illness.

Some food may give you energy, but it's important to be mindful of the quality of energy that food gives you. Sugar tends to provide wiry energy, while complex carbohydrates such as whole grains give a more sustained energy. Avoid foods that feel like they sit like a rock in your stomach; the energy your body is using to digest them may be greater than the nutrients that the food offers.

By following these ten steps to healthy eating, you may not only become healthier, but may also begin to appreciate the food you eat. Eating to live may eventually be more important and enjoyable than living to eat.

7

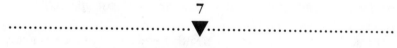

USE IT OR LOSE IT

The only reason I would take up jogging is so that I could hear heavy breathing again.
Erma Bombeck

Not long ago a typical person felt a strong urge to rest after a hard day's work. In today's sedentary times, after a hard day's work you're more apt to feel a strong urge to exercise.

Exercise is considered an essential ingredient for maintaining and enhancing a person's overall state of health. Exercise is certainly a helpful factor in improving cardiovascular and respiratory health, maintaining overall muscle tone, and aiding weight control. Exercise alone, however, is not adequate to maintain health, as has been evidenced by the early deaths of many professional and Olympic athletes.

Exercise plays an even larger role in health than these common areas of concern. Most people don't know, for instance, that before the discovery of insulin, physical activity was the primary therapy for diabetes mellitus. Although exercise alone will not cure diabetes, research has shown that physical activity does allow the diabetic to reduce insulin dosages.

Exercise is also a treatment recommended by a growing number of psychiatrists and psychologists for healing depression. When you consider that some people do not want to risk exercising without first obtaining a doctor's permission, there is enough evidence to support its value to suggest that one should seek medical permission if you do not wish to exercise. With the side effects of exercise being a healthier heart, firmer muscles, slimmer figure, and a more positive disposition, more therapists should become coaches . . . and visa versa.

It's been proven that if a person maintains the same caloric intake for one year and simply increases his activity level by walking one mile per day, that person would lose approximately ten pounds of fat tissue.

In addition to the various health benefits of exercise, many people exercise simply because it feels good. Some people even report that they get high when they exercise. Evidence has shown that physical activity releases endorphins which are the body's natural painkillers. These opiate-like chemicals actually create a sense of being high; research suggests that some people even become addicted to this feeling. I'm certainly not suggesting you go that far; the point is that exercise can make you feel great at the same time that it's doing great things for your body.

The biggest obstacle that keeps most people from regular exercise is discipline. Perhaps they think that discipline means denying themselves something. It doesn't have to be. The best way to discipline yourself is to simply remember what you want; what you *really* want. If, for instance, you really want to lose fifteen pounds, by focusing on this goal and by reminding yourself of the pleasure that you will get from losing this weight, you will be less distracted by obstacles, and the goal becomes more attainable.

Try to do an activity once a day to get yourself out of breath for at least fifteen minutes. (Making love doesn't count. Fortunately, for most people, "use it or lose it" doesn't apply to such indoor sports.) Choose exercises that you really enjoy, otherwise you won't stick with them. Jogging, swimming, weight-lifting, aerobics, and certain competitive sports build muscular strength and cardiovascular health, while other exercises such as yoga, dance, and various martial arts help to build balance, flexibility, and coordination of mind and body. Make exercise a part of your everyday life and do those little things to encourage it: take stairs instead of an elevator, ride your bike for simple chores instead of driving a car, and use a manual lawnmower.

This bit of health wisdom about the once-a-day activity applies to mental exercise as well. Just as you may go to a gym or playing field to exercise, you should also perform mental workouts. There are innumerable everyday mental exercises that you can do to improve your memory, comprehension, concentration, and creativity. You can, for instance, make a greater effort to remember people's names and their phone numbers. You can read a newspaper and then several hours later describe to a friend the stories you read, with your own commentary on them. Your concentration can be exercised by meditating for twenty minutes and doing your best to avoid thinking of anything else. You can exercise your own creativity by composing a poem, cooking an exotic dish without a recipe, or rearranging the furniture in your home.

If you don't exercise your mind, stretching it and challenging it regularly, it will become lazy and limp. Just as physically lazy people will become breathless from simple exertion, mentally lazy people can go blank in simple conversation. This may explain why people who suffer from couch potato-itis are not only physically out of shape, they are often unable to carry on a serious conversation.

Some people who suffer from couch potato-itis may actually seem very intelligent. They are often excellent at Trivial Pursuit, (thanks to "Jeopardy") and they may be great at Scrabble (thanks to "Wheel of Fortune"). But don't be fooled by this—they may be TV-smart but intellect-foolish.

So, remember to exercise your body *and* your mind. Considering all the value received from exercising, it is surprising that it isn't taxed.

8

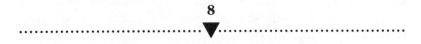

OPENING NATURE'S MEDICINE CABINET

A weed is an herb whose virtue has not yet been recognized.
Ralph Waldo Emerson

As any gardener knows, weeds can be hardy plants and not easy to eliminate from a garden. Perhaps this very persistence constitutes their virtue as well. A weed's ability to grow and even flourish in the smallest crack in the cement shows a certain strength and flexibility. One may wonder if strength and flexibility, given the choice of the right weed, is inevitably transfered to a sick person who ingests it.

Every culture throughout time has used and even relied upon herbal preparations. In teas, in poultices, in foods, or simply in their raw state, herbs have been found to heal and prevent disease. (Like every healing system, however, one has to learn how to use them properly, for some herbs are harmful if overused and others are poisonous even if ingested in relatively small amounts.)

Herbs are even beginning to be used by a growing number of physicians—finally. Since many conventional drugs are actually derived from herbs, it makes sense to cut out the middleman—

22

the drug companies—and go directly to the source. Not only is it cheaper, it's safer.

Whereas drug companies only tend to utilize the most powerful ingredient of an herb, there are often other important ingredients in an herb that are not included in the drug. These other ingredients often help the body metabolize the primary ingredient and sometimes even protect people from poisoning themselves. The herb foxglove, *Digitalis purpurea*, for instance, contains a heart stimulant—digitoxin—which is used in the drug by this name, but it also contains a heart depressant—digitonin. Perhaps this is nature's balancing act, its way of making it more difficult for humans and other animals to harm themselves. Interestingly, another ingredient in foxglove which is not in the conventional drug derived from it is a compound that causes nausea and vomiting, symptoms that warn an unsuspecting user that he is taking too much of the herb, thus helping to protect him from ingesting an amount that may adversely affect the heart.

If drug companies could patent herbs, they would certainly sponsor more research to discover their value. Many herbs have already been found to have strong antibacterial and antiviral properties. Others have been found to have antitumor capability, and still others have been shown to reduce cholesterol and blood pressure. But because herbal medicine does not presently have significant governmental or corporate support sponsoring research or public educational efforts, the public and the medical community remain largely ignorant of its real value.

There's no need for you to be, though. You'll find it worthwhile to cultivate a good relationship with these valuable substances. An herb is a terrible thing to waste.

9

▼

THE HAIR OF THE DOG THAT BITES YOU HEALS YOU

To like things like,
whatever one may ail,
there is certain help.
Johann Wolfgang von Goethe

The folk saying about the hair of the dog is an ancient bit of wisdom and an integral part of modern medicine as well.

According to Greek mythology, Apollo proclaimed through the Oracle at Delphi "that which makes sick shall heal." When the Greek hero Telephus was speared, he needed to apply the original spear to his injury to heal himself. This treating of like with like was also commonly used by the Mayans, Chinese, and many ancient peoples. Treating wasp bites with a compound made of the crushed nests of wasps, and healing jaundice with yellow herbs such as celendine are but two examples of this ancient principle of pharmacology.

The use of "like" to treat "like" is also an integral part of conventional medicine today, as witnessed in the use of immunizations and allergy treatments. Immunizations usually consist of small doses of bacteria or viruses that cause an infection in order to stimulate an immune response that will prevent a more serious infection. Likewise, allergy treatments use small doses of an allergen to strengthen the adaptive capacities of the body so that it no longer reacts to the substance hypersensitively.

Despite these rare uses of like to treat like in conventional medicine, more commonly physicians use drugs that have an opposite action on the person's symptoms. For instance, a person with constipation will be given a laxative, and a person with diarrhea is given something that constipates him. A person with an inactive thyroid gland will be given a thyroid hormone, and a person with an overactive thyroid gland will be given a drug to inhibit excess secretion of its hormone.

However, the inherent assumption behind the use of opposites in treating sick people is that their body is doing something wrong or that it doesn't know what it is doing. In contrast, the use of similars in treating sick people recognizes that there's an inherent wisdom of the body and a defensive value of its symptoms. Instead of inhibiting this response, using medicines that augment the body's inherent healing capacities promotes real healing, not simply symptom suppression.

Homeopathic medicine is a pharmaceutical science that is entirely based on treating like with like. It uses small doses of substances which have the capacity, when given in overdose, to cause a pattern of symptoms similar to what the sick person is experiencing. The homeopathic physician's application of the law of similars is, however, distinct from the conventional physician's application of it. Homeopaths use considerably smaller doses of these potentially poisonous substances, and they individualize the prescription to a much more significant degree, taking into account the entire range of the patient's symptoms, not simply making a generic prescription for a generic disease.

Indeed, one of the challenges of using homeopathy is figuring out the appropriate remedy for each ailment. Because the most effective way to apply the remedies is to tailor their prescription to a person's unique pattern of symptoms, there is rarely one medicine for everybody's problem. One person's form of arthritis, headache, or allergy is often distinct from another person's similar problem, and requires a treatment that addresses those distinctions.

A person with arthritis may experience much swelling in the joints along with burning and stinging pains which feels worse with heat and better with cold application. The person may be awkward, clumsy, and have a tendency to drop things. He may have little or no thirst and in general may be sensitive to touch.

This pattern of symptoms can be caused by bee venom (*Apis*) in healthy people and can also be healed with homeopathic doses of it.

Using a substance that actually *causes* arthritis symptoms to treat them may sound strange; however, because symptoms of illness are adaptive responses of the organism to stress or infection, the use of a substance similar to what causes the problem makes sense since this treatment helps to augment the body's natural defensive efforts. Rather than using drugs to suppress symptoms, the law of similars gently and safely aids in the body's own effort to heal itself.

There are numerous books on homeopathy—and even computer software—available to help you determine which remedies to use in which situations. This book too provides some broad guidelines for its application.

Keep in mind that there are right and wrong ways to make use of the law of similars. Do not attempt to treat a pounding headache with a hammer, or try to treat a broken leg by breaking the other leg. And don't treat a barking cough with a hair of your pet dog. The principle of similars can be a powerful healing tool, but like any tool, you must know how to use it.

10

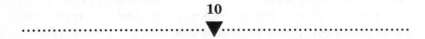

A LITTLE DAB WILL DO YA

Little by little does the trick.
Aesop

According to the military's version of Humpty Dumpty, after Humpty fell, the General asserted, "All the King's horses and all the King's men couldn't put Humpty together again. Therefore, I'm going to need more horses and more men."

Conventional medical solutions tend to be like military solutions. Too often, physicians assert that stronger medicine or more sophisticated medical technology is the answer to illness. Sometimes, the best solution is to stop all treatment and let the person's personal doctor—his own body—do its own work.

The human organism already knows how to heal itself; often it doesn't need the big guns of medicine, but can adequately and effectively heal itself using less biologically disruptive strategies. When small changes occur in certain key biological systems, they create a significant cascade effect on other systems, eventually leading to major changes. There are, for instance, numerous substances that can, in small doses, stimulate the production of certain enzymes which will then stimulate liver, kidney, or heart function, which in turn affects every system and cell of the body.

Rather than overwhelm the body with powerful drugs or with mega-doses of vitamins, it is sometimes more effective to just nudge the healing process along gently. A small dose of the proper nutrient, a single stimulus to the appropriate acupuncture point, a catalyst from a well-chosen herb, or an individualized application of a small dose of a homeopathic medicine may be all that is necessary to initiate the healing process.

Homeopathic medicine is a classic example of a medical therapy where less is more. Homeopathy uses extremely small doses of substances which, when individually prescribed to a person's unique pattern of symptoms, have the capacity to stimulate deep healing. It's not that small doses of any substance will work; it's small doses of a *key substance* that can catalyze significant reactions.

Another example is using light as a treatment for the body. It is widely known in medicine that the amount and type of light we absorb affects our brain chemistry and hormonal patterns. Even psychiatrists acknowledge the existence of *winter depression*—a condition created by lack of sunlight and treated with doses of light. Because sometimes less is more, this treatment does not consist of one hundred spotlights overwhelming the sick person but of a couple of low wattage, full-spectrum lights for an hour or two a day.

The use of small doses of a specific therapy does not necessarily preclude the value of large doses. Conventional drugs or megadoses of vitamins and minerals have their place in health care, particularly in treating certain infections or in advanced pathology. However, large doses, especially of certain drugs, are potentially dangerous.

What is most problematic about large doses of medicine is their tendency to create new symptoms. Although there is a tendency to call these symptoms *side effects*, this is actually a misnomer. We arbitrarily differentiate those effects of a drug that we like from those that we don't like, and we then call the latter—the new symptoms—side effects. More precisely, these new symptoms are the result of the drug suppressing the person's present symptoms, or are simply the body's reaction to the drug's toxic ingredients. Small doses, on the other hand, do not generally carry these dangers, which is a safety factor that should be taken more seriously by physicians today. Strategies that recognize the value and the power of small doses represent a healthy respect for the human organism. Once you realize that the human body has an inherent wisdom, you understand that doing something major to it only tends to hinder the body from doing it itself. Using small doses of treatment, on the other hand, gently nudges the body in the direction that it knows it must go.

The body knows how to heal itself. It has been doing it for a long long time. Our job is not to try to take over its job.

11

................................▼................................

SOME OF MY BEST FRIENDS ARE GERMS

Each new antibiotic brings into being literally millions of microscopic Benedict Arnolds.
Marc Lappe, Ph.D.

Like a Hollywood movie with good guys and bad guys, the human body plays out its daily soap opera helped by the "good" bacteria and struggling against "bad" bacteria. The good bacteria play an instrumental part in aiding our digestion of food; they appear on the skin and oral cavity, help to fight infection by creating their own natural antibiotics, and have been found to stimulate the immune system by serving as a low-level "tonic." The bad bacteria, on the other hand, grow wherever and whenever conditions are favorable for them and cause inflammation, pain, and sometimes death.

There are anywhere from a hundred thousand to one million of these microscopic organisms on each square centimeter of your skin. There are actually ten times this amount on areas of the skin which are moist for prolonged periods of time. The webs of the toes, for instance, often carry tens of millions of bacteria of diverse kinds. In total, there are approximately *one trillion* bacteria on our skin alone, and there are perhaps *one hundred trillion* more inside the body. Although some people may be horrified to discover that we are literally surrounded by bacteria inside and out, it is important to remember that many of these bacteria not only provide the essential benefits to the body mentioned earlier, but they also help produce vitamin K, biotin, riboflavin, pyridoxine, and other vitamins essential for bodily function. Bacteria have definitely been given a bum rap. We wouldn't be here without them.

Still, certain types of bacteria can lead to illness in people who are susceptible to them. Streptococcus can invade the throat, pneumococcus can infiltrate lung tissue, and gonococcus can infect mucous membranes. People with bacterial infections are commonly prescribed antibiotics like ampicillin, tetracyline, amoxicillin, or others. Although these antibiotics, with their infection-fighting abilities, can be literally lifesaving, they can also be the cause of many problems; they do not just attack the bad guys but too often get the good guys too. And unlike a Hollywood movie, the good guys don't always win in the end.

Despite the power of antibiotics, bacteria are often strong enough and smart enough to outwit and outfight them. Once an antibiotic kills a bacteria's friend or relative, the bacteria wants to get even; it quickly learns to adapt to the antibiotic and develop a resistance to it. This is why different and stronger antibiotics are often necessary for treating bacterial infections. This is also why Harvard professor and Nobel Prize-winner Walter Gilbert has predicted that sometime in the future 80 to 90 percent of infections will be resistant to all known antibiotics.

The use of antibiotics can lead to many long-term health problems. Antibiotics not only knock out the good bacteria with the bad, but also create a more favorable environment for various yeast infections, from such opportunists as *Candida albicans*, which leads to vaginitis and numerous other chronic health problems, to *Clostridium difficile*, which leads to colitis.

The use of antibiotics to treat infections can be likened to the farmer who tries insecticides to rid his swamp of mosquitoes. The insecticide kills the mosquitoes, but the swamp is still a swamp, and a breeding ground for a new infestation. Instead of attacking the mosquito, more holistic and ecological solutions would be to drain the swamp or bring in frogs that eat mosquito eggs.

Likewise, rather than attacking the bacteria with antibiotics, it may be more effective to consider various natural therapies that strengthen your immune system, thereby improving your body's ability to defend itself. Various herbs, including licorice root and echinacea, certain foods such as shiitake mushrooms and garlic, and individualized treatments of homeopathic medicines and acupuncture have all been shown to stimulate immune response. Also, methods that calm, energize, or balance your emotional and mental state may be valuable. Louis Pasteur, as well as many other physicians and scientists, suggested that a person's psychological state could influence resistance to microbes. Meditation, relaxation, and various other stress-management approaches are potentially effective strategies to both prevent and treat certain infectious conditions.

Despite the value of these alternatives, at times antibiotics are still the most effective way to heal certain infections. But just because you are using antibiotics doesn't mean that you should ignore natural therapies. In fact, one way to reduce their possible side effects is to take acidophilus—one of the friendly types of intestinal bacteria—available in pill form, or in yogurt or miso. By replenishing your intestines with this beneficial bacteria, you may not only feel better sooner, you may be less likely to get reinfected.

Making matters a bit more complicated, however, are the actions of a majority of American farmers, who feed huge amounts of antibiotics to their chickens, pigs, and cows as a way to prevent infection. When we eat the meat, milk, or eggs of these animals, we also ingest trace amounts of these antibiotics. Many scientists have suggested that these small amounts enable the harmful bacteria in us to adapt to larger medicinal doses of antibiotics. Because of this, conventional doses of antibiotics may not work as well for us, and more powerful doses or stronger antibiotics become increasingly necessary.

Native American Chief Seattle wisely warned Western civilization of the problems inherent in ignoring the interrelationships of life when he said, "We are part of the web of life. We are not the weaver. When a part of the web is destroyed, a part of ourselves is hurt." Although he was referring to the way we understand and treat our environment, his words also have meaning for our internal environment, our bodies.

As much as we may boo and hiss when the bad bacteria enter the picture, they should not simply be considered the villains.

They alert us to a personal weakness that has enabled the bacteria to grow, they can challenge and ultimately strengthen our immune system, and they encourage a microbial diversity that can actually lead to biological stability.

This information is not meant to imply that antibiotics aren't valuable, lifesaving drugs. However, it is absolutely vital that we use antibiotics judiciously. We should use alternatives first and resort to these drugs in medical emergencies.

12

MAKE FRIENDS WITH YOUR PAIN

*Sometimes your pain doesn't make your life unbearable;
your life makes your pain unbearable.*
David Bresler, Ph.D.

The word *pain* is derived from the Latin word *poena* which means punishment. Whether pain should be thought of as a punishment is debatable, but we know that it certainly hurts to have it, and it usually feels like a punishment, whether we feel like we've done something to deserve it or not. In ancient times people thought that pain was caused by demons who had possessed them. Anyone who has experienced much pain can easily understand this point of view.

Pain is nature's way of getting your attention. It is a warning that something is wrong. It is a symptom and a signal, and it demands your attention—often too much of your attention.

Headaches, backaches, arthritis, and menstrual cramps are the most commonly experienced pain syndromes. As much as most people in pain try to get rid of it, methods that simply suppress pain do not heal the cause and can drive the pain deeper. Most people treat their pain with one or more of the various anti-inflammatory medicines, also known as painkillers. However, because pain itself is only a symptom, painkillers may reduce the discomfort experienced, but they do nothing to heal the source of pain. In fact, the body eventually adapts to the painkillers and soon needs stronger and stronger doses in order to achieve a similar degree of relief. The body also becomes addicted to these drugs, ultimately causing new types of discomforts and dysfunctions which you might want to treat with additional drugs. A pain cycle has been created, and it is sometimes difficult to break it.

Denying pain is equally ineffective and can be very dangerous. Some people ignore their pain. They insist that nothing is wrong, that there is nothing that they should change about themselves, and that the pain they are having is only a temporary glitch that will soon disappear.

The famed psychiatrist Carl Jung once said, "If you don't come to terms with your shadow, it will appear in your life as your fate." Until you come to terms with your pain, its fateful return will be a continual reminder of something wrong. It has been said that "denial ain't just a river in Egypt." Denial runs deep and wide, but you cannot wash away your pain by ignoring it. Until awareness replaces denial, the pain will simply keep demanding attention one way or another.

The challenge of pain is to understand what it is saying. What is it in your life that is not in balance? Is there something that you need to change within yourself, or is there something outside that needs to be avoided or changed? Does the location and kind of pain have any special meaning to you? And why did the pain begin now?

Whatever the source of pain, it represents a certain wisdom of the body and mind to defend themselves against stress or infection. Whatever the nature of the pain, it is decidely safer and more effective to appreciate it rather than resist it. Resistance creates additional tension and usually additional pain, while loving attention can have a noticeably soothing and healing effect.

Loving your pain is certainly easier to say than to do. It seems a lot easier to feel irritated and angry about the pain, depressed and despairing about how horrible it is, and fearful and anxious about how long the pain will go on. But just as you can act as if life is just a series of problems, you can also be challenged by life as a series of adventures. Instead of fretting about the pain, you can be creatively seeking out ways to deal with it.

There is also something wonderfully healing when you simply give pain positive vibrations. Although this may sound hokey, when you're in pain you're usually willing to do some pretty odd things get relief. Since fighting pain is like pulling at a knot from both ends, learning to love and play with the knot sometimes loosens its grip.

As heroes in many a fairytale have shown, "You don't have to hate the dragon to love the princess." Likewise, you don't have to hate the pain to love the challenge that it creates. This may be an important first step in learning to deal with pain most effectively.

13

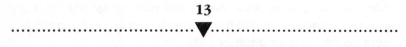

TAKE LAUGHTER SERIOUSLY

You don't stop laughing because you grow old; you grow old because you stop laughing.
Michael Prichard

When faced with adversity, most species choose fight or flight. Humans, however, have a third choice: to laugh. A good laugh reduces tension. Finding humor in a stressful situation often diffuses it. Many people don't take laughter seriously. They think that it's kid's stuff or unprofessional or simply inappropriate, considering all of the world's problems. And yet humor and laughter are integral parts of our humanness; they can give us a different and healthier perspective on a problem. They can break the ice and create a more trusting relationship. They may also create a sense of joy so that even if you are defeated or in pain, joy and its memories will provide a healing salve.

It is not simply a coincidence that laughter is said to "break you up"; it stimulates a healthy internal jogging. As with actual jogging, laughter promotes faster and deeper breathing, greater oxygen supply throughout the bloodstream, and increased heart rate and blood pressure. Vigorous and frequent laughter can even help to burn up as many calories as many common physical activities. Studies have even shown that merely smiling creates beneficial changes in body chemistry, even when the smile is faked. The curved line of a smile indeed sometimes straightens everything out.

Humor and laughter are especially important when you are ill. Laughter has been shown to improve immune function and increase your ability to withstand pain. And the only side effect of this treatment is joyful memories. Although you might say "it hurts when I laugh," more often it hurts when you don't.

Unfortunately, it seems that the majority of physicians and scientists are more interested in studying the negative emotional states that may lead to disease rather than studying those positive emotional states that may lead to healthier and happier people. But even the Bible acknowledges that "A merry heart doeth good like a medicine" (Proverbs 17:22). Perhaps doctors in the future will be as likely to prescribe Robin Williams, Woody Allen, or Marx Brothers movies as they are to prescribe drugs.

Laughter is just as infective as germs, and can be wonderfully contagious. It will rarely cure you on its own, but it sure will make your problems more bearable. As the saying goes, angels can fly because they take themselves lightly.

Laughter is not just a temporary bandage; it is good long-term medicine. Studies have shown that people who are hopeful and optimistic tend to live longer and healthier lives. Perhaps the saying should be changed to "he who laughs, *lasts*."

Not only does laughter feel good, it is good for you. Have you had your minimum daily dose today?

14
▼

RELAX, BUT APPRECIATE STRESS

Stress is the spice of life.
Complete freedom from stress is death.
Hans Selye, M.D.

Everybody is always telling us to relax. If you're depressed about something that just happened, relax. If you're worried about something in the future, relax. Even if you're extremely excited about something, someone is bound to tell you to relax.

Sounds great, but the goal of life is more than feeling relaxed. And what's worse is that if you relax too much, you may turn into mush.

Stress has become the bad guy. We are supposed to avoid it, reduce it, and manage it. It seems that stress is being blamed for nearly everything. Actually, stress is an integral part of life and living. The Chinese character for the word *crisis* is actually a combination of two words: danger and opportunity. Stress, also, is a sign of danger and an opportunity to grow. Although stress can lead to discomfort and disease, it can also be seen as a challenge that can make you stronger.

Stress only becomes a problem when there is too much of it to make good use of it. Just as the body gets fatigued from overwork, so does the brain. The brain can burn as many calories during intense concentration or great anxiety as do muscles during exercise. Perhaps weight-loss farms of the future will have chess games instead of aerobics classes. However, thinking too much can be exhausting and too many emotional experiences can be draining: that's where relaxation can be helpful.

The initial stages of relaxation can be relatively easy. Sitting or laying down comfortably in a quiet environment, closing your eyes, and breathing deeply and slowly, are important in achieving some degree of relaxation. The initial stages of relaxation enable you to slow down and literally catch your breath.

However, frequent or distressing thoughts all too often rush to the forefront of one's mind. There are various strategies for dealing with this mental chatter, and some people devote their lives to perfecting their ability to create an inner calm. Some focus on their breathing, others on their mantra (a phrase that is continually repeated), and still others on a pleasant or pleasurable feeling or experience they have had.

Another strategy for dealing with incessant mental chatter is to try to let go of any and all thoughts as they arise. If they return, let them go again, avoid trying to solve problems during this time, and simply *be*, without trying to think anything, feel anything, or do anything. Interestingly, thinking, feeling, and doing nothing is much harder than you would think.

Although you might certainly wonder how and why doing nothing can be of any benefit, a growing body of scientific evidence has begun to confirm the therapeutic value of deep relaxation. Besides lowering blood pressure, deep relaxation can also stimulate the body's immune system. It is almost as though relaxation helps us get out of the way of the body's inherent self-healing capacities. Just as the body is more able to heal itself during sleep, conscious relaxation provides the body with a great opportunity for healing.

Learning to relax is one important strategy, but like every strategy, it has its limitations.

Relaxing does little to stop your inappropriate behavior or that of others. Relaxing does nothing to improve relationships. And relaxation does not solve the various problems outside of you that may be the whole reason you need to relax in the first place.

Relaxation is invaluable for getting to that centered place within, to that inner sense of peace and security, but unless you act from this relaxed point in a purposeful manner, relaxation only becomes an escape, not a way to resolve a bad situation.

So ... relax, but don't turn into mush.

15

▼

IT'S THE LITTLE THINGS THAT GET YOU

Rule #1 is, don't sweat the small stuff. Rule #2 is, it's all small stuff. And if you can't fight and you can't flee, flow.
R. S. Eliot

We all know that major stresses in our lives, such as deaths in the family, divorces, or tax audits, can have a significant impact on our health. However, the accumulation of smaller stresses, especially when recurrent and prolonged, can have a similar significant, detrimental effect. The stress felt driving in rush-hour traffic, or talking to a person who is being difficult, dealing with various family problems, or keeping a home clean and organized every day adds wrinkles to our faces, anxieties to our stomachs, and wobbles to our knees. These extra weights are sometimes enough to topple us when we are doing everything we can to maintain life's balancing act.

A tyrannical executive was once asked if he had high blood pressure. He said, "No, but I'm a carrier." All too often employers, friends, or even strangers do things that not only stress others but aggravate an underlying problem that had been lying dormant. A little stress can set off a chain reaction. The mouse is roaring.

Little problems add up to create major problems unless they are dealt with as they occur. The mind has a natural tendency to try to work out stressful experiences. Dangling situations obscure our vision of the world and force us to re-experience those situations until they are made right. Our dreams and nightmares commonly become the theater in which the leftover dramas of our daily life are replayed.

One way to deal with the small day-to-day stresses is, first of all, to know that they are there. Once you realize that you are experiencing subtle and sometimes not so subtle stresses, you can decide to do something about them. The following techniques may be helpful.

Head them off at the pass

Prevent the little stresses by first anticipating and then avoiding them. Determine what your most common little stresses are and do whatever is necessary to avoid them or deal with them as they develop. If, for instance, you have to drive in rush-hour traffic, listen to an enjoyable tape while you drive. If you are dealing with a difficult person daily, try to diffuse their negativity by being nice to them.

Do a body-check

At least once a day do this exercise: close your eyes and move your consciousness to various parts of your body, looking for areas that feel stiff or stuck. Shake the area, massage it, breathe into it, and then relax it. Consider how and why a particular part of your body is stiff or stuck. You may find you can shake off the minor stresses right along with the stiffness.

Do a life-check

Just as many people have "to do" lists in their daily life, it is helpful to have a life-check list: assess how you are doing, what barriers are in the way of where you want to be, and how you plan to get over or around them.

We usually focus on the big problems in our lives and try to figure out what to do about them. Too often we neglect to see how the small things add up to create big problems.

▼

16

SELF-MEDICATE WITH SELF-ESTEEM

If you put a small value upon yourself, rest assured that the world will not raise the price.
Anonymous

How you feel about yourself may actually affect the way your body defends itself against the stresses and infective organisms that surround it. During infection, the body's white blood cells identify foreign microorganisms and then work to devour them. The body's ability to identify its own cells from those of foreign organisms or substances is vital for healthy functioning.

But just as you may sometimes experience an identity crisis, the body at times has difficulty differentiating itself from foreign life forms. Without this ability to detect self from non-self you are prone to infection and disease. Since the body and mind are inexorably connected, it seems feasible that low self-esteem—a diminished sense of identity—can also damage immune function.

On the other hand, a high level of self-esteem, or a stronger sense of self, could lead to a more vigorous immune response. While this doesn't mean that people with high self-esteem will never get sick, it does mean that they will probably be better equipped to deal with whatever stresses or diseases they encounter.

Each threat to your health can strengthen your ability to survive. Each symptom of disease, though painful and discomforting, is a result of your body's best effort to respond to stress or infection. Likewise, each doubt about yourself can be approached as a challenge. Each doubt, like each symptom, can be an important personal defense and a potentially helpful lesson on how to live in the world.

Developing high self-esteem is particularly difficult if you've been continually told that you're a loser. It is helpful to know, however, that a winner in self-esteem is rarely a born winner, but is often someone who is successful because of the blood, sweat, and years he has committed to a goal. Self-esteem is not even necessarily linked to winning or losing; rather, each experience is seen as an opportunity to gain greater self-knowledge and a richer sense of life-awareness. It's not important to win; it's important to learn and grow.

For instance, the first white man to scale Mt. Everest failed on his first two tries. After the second try, he addressed his sponsors, the Board of Directors of the National Geographic Society. Rather than berate himself or apologize for his failures, he simply showed them a picture of Mt. Everest and said, "This mountain will never grow another inch, but with each failure, I learn and I grow." On his third attempt, he reached the top.

If you fail at something or if people call you a loser, it is indeed easy to feel terrible about yourself, get depressed, or become ill. The sickness cycle is created when you feel unhappy and insecure, and then become more depressed now that you are ill.

The way out of this cycle may sound trite, but it's true: we need to remind ourselves that we are all really winners. When you think about it, each of our fathers created millions and millions of sperm, each of our mothers created egg after egg after egg . . . and *we* were the ones that made it!

Another way out of the loser/illness cycle is to try to move beyond the winner/loser mentality. Life is not a contest with winners and losers. Competition may be appropriate for animals in the wild or for baseball and football players, but it is not a necessary ingredient for living in today's civilized society.

Self-esteem cannot be given to you, or be bought, sold, or traded. If you try to base it solely on material success, personal appearance, fame, or occupation, these transient and superficial factors provide only a temporary and often false sense of self-value. And if you pretend to have self-esteem, you just fool yourself. Ultimately, your life and your health become your own lie detector test.

Self-esteem is inevitably an inside job, and this good feeling deep inside yourself radiates outward, creating a healthier body and a state of contagious good vibes.

Don't just stand there, full esteem ahead.

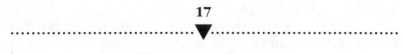

17

FOLLOW YOUR BLISS

*Dwell as near as possible to the channel
in which your life flows.*
Henry David Thoreau

"Be Here Now" was a personal and spiritual motto of many people in the 1970s; "Follow Your Bliss" is taking its place in the 1990s. "Follow Your Bliss" means to discover and act upon that which gives your life meaning. It means doing things to which you are somehow drawn. It does not mean simply doing things that give you pleasure; it means following the yearnings of your heart, your mind, your very soul.

"Take your passion and make it happen" are words from the title song in the movie *Flashdance.* Like "Follow Your Bliss," these words encourage you to do those things that are truly important, even vital, to you. Just as food feeds the body, living your passion is food for the soul. Such soul food is *real* health food.

When people have purpose and meaning in their life, it is amazing how much they can endure to attain their goal. There are innumerable examples of people overcoming their devastating pain or life-threatening illness in order to finish their important work. Your work might be anything—from caring for your children to painting a picture, writing a book, or healing others.

Meaning and purpose in your life can be found in your family, job, community, or personal growth; whatever it is, it directly affects your health. A United States government study, for instance, showed that the most important factor in good health was not a person's diet, exercise, or stress management, but the degree of work satisfaction. Although this information may surprise some people, it will make complete sense to others. Not only do many people spend more time at work than anywhere else, but many people's personal identity, self-worth, and sense of community are an integral part of their job. Their job is not simply what they do to make money, it is also their connection and contribution to the world. To fortunate people, their job is an important part of their mission in life as well.

While you may take the time to conscientiously relax for thirty minutes a day, the five to ten hours of work you do each day have a much greater and enduring effect on your life and health. It is no wonder that it is healthier to take your job and love it than it is to take it and ... Indeed, having work that you love can be one of the most powerful healing strategies.

Perhaps it is no accident that the word *vocation* is derived from a Latin word which means "a calling." Whether your calling is your work or not, having a mission in life creates the ability to shine light into whatever darkness you may be experiencing. Doing what you love creates a special happiness and a unique connectedness to others, the result of the heartful efforts that are being made.

Following your bliss allows bliss to follow you. Not only do people who have a sense of purpose in life often seem more happy within themselves, they also radiate a contagious aliveness that infects those around them.

Although people who are following their bliss eventually die just like everyone else, their quality of life is significantly different. Sometimes this improved quality of life improves your health, but perhaps more importantly, this improved health helps you to further achieve your life purpose.

While most people hope to attain whatever their life's goal is, it is not as important to be successful as it is to try heartfully. This is when you know that you are doing your life's work: when you are so involved and so clear and certain about your mission that the process of getting there is in itself fulfilling.

Having a calling, mission, or goal in your life helps give you direction. Rather than simply floating aimlessly from one experience to another, with a direction you are going somewhere, and mysteriously enough, when you have a direction you are often directed; you are somehow guided and aided in your efforts.

Such is the mystery of life. How now, great Tao.

18

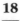

THE POWER OF PRAYER IS GREATER THAN YOU THINK

Every time I pray to God,
I find that I am talking to myself.
Peter O'Toole

You do not have to clasp your hands together in order to pray. Every thought is a prayer. Every thought creates biochemical processes that subtly and sometimes significantly change the way you are. Simply visualizing or wishing for something can be the first step to making it happen.

The most powerful prayers, however, are more than just thinking, visualizing, or wishing. They are profound expressions of the soul's desires, or deep expressions of gratitude.

People commonly pray for health, either for others or for themselves, and research has shown that prayer can have significant healing effects. Whether it's because an outside force helps the person heal or because of the healing love that the person experiences from themselves or others, prayer can work.

To whom or what one prays seems to be secondary to the act of praying. For every person who says that his God is the most effective healer, there are others who say the same thing about their God. And for every person who claims that an external force has healed them, there are others who believe that the healing came from within. One belief system is probably no more valid than the other, for if this force is as all-pervading as most people claim, perhaps everyone is talking about the same force, but using different names.

A prayer usually contains a goal, an image, and a profound desire for something to happen, but you must also be willing to accept whatever happens, to surrender to the truth, and to the selflessness of love behind the prayer in order for the prayer to have the best chance to work its wonders.

As we think and wish and pray, we create the initial building blocks that lead to action. A thought or prayer is the Pavlov's bell that gets a person salivating for what he wants. Once this salivation begins, the hunger must lead to action. Just because you're hungry doesn't mean you'll get fed. A thought or prayer will lie dormant unless you act to achieve it or put yourself in a position to receive what you're asking for.

As some people believe, Determination + Prayer + Action = Result. Without the determination and action, prayer alone usually remains visualization without manifestation.

Praying for health requires a certain non-attachment to the goal. A woman, for instance, may pray for relief from her headache, but if she is extremely anxious in her prayers, this anxiety can impede healing. Likewise, a father may pray so desperately for his sick child that his fears may be felt by the child and interfere with the potential for healing.

You must be careful what you pray for; you might get it ... literally.

The good news (and the bad news) about prayer is that you often get much more than you pray for. Like the athlete who prayed for less pain in his sprained ankle but then injured it more seriously when trying to go back to competition too early. Or like the person who prayed for less severe psoriasis symptoms, but then developed a more painful arthritic condition. One must remember that whatever you pray for, you also get the baggage that comes with it.

A certain amount of clarity, openness, persistence, and trust can always improve your chances for getting prayers answered. However, whether you get what you are praying for or not, it would be wise to keep in mind the words of the Rolling Stones: "You can't always get what you want, but if you try sometimes, you just might find you get what you need."

19

▼

EVERYBODY IS A GRANDMOTHER

He who neglects to drink of the spring of experience is likely to die of thirst in the desert of ignorance.

Ling Po

Everybody is a grandmother because everyone has her or his own sage advice and personal experience. Although Will Rogers once said, "Everybody is ignorant, just on different subjects," the opposite of this statement is also true: everybody is an expert, just on different subjects.

We all have our own experience of what healing techniques work and what don't. Simply living forty years means that a person has experienced forty cold and flu seasons, eighty allergy seasons (spring and fall), and innumerable stomachaches, headaches, coughs, and injuries.

After forty years of successful and unsuccessful treatments of these various problems, everybody has some special strategies. This becomes obvious when you catch a simple cold: people will inevitably tell you what *they* do when they have a cold.

We too often give more credence to professionals with a degree than to people with experience. This logic was classically demonstrated when the Wizard in *The Wizard of Oz* gave the Scarecrow a diploma instead of a brain. The Scarecrow accepted it as a sufficient substitute. We too often assume that a diploma means brains.

But the best knowledge comes from experience. It has been said: "Tell me, and I will forget. Show me, and I will try to understand. Let me do it, and I will learn." Experience gives us the opportunity of involvement, and it gives us a chance to receive real knowledge. Ultimately though, experience is not what happens to you; it is what you do with what happens to you.

One problem with using experience as a guide is that the final exam often comes first and is then followed by the lesson. Ralph Waldo Emerson seemed to understand this paradox when he said, "Life is a succession of lessons which must be lived to be understood."

If you do not have the experience yourself, seek others who may have it. Such people are often older than you are, though not always. It is usually preferred to heed the advice of those who have come out the other side of the experience rather than those who are experts in living with the problem, though any experience carries its own wisdom on how to do something . . . or how *not* to do it.

Knowledge and wisdom does not simply come from positive experiences. As Senator Bob Packwood once said, "Judgment comes from experience, and great judgment comes from bad experience."

Learning from another's experience can be helpful but can also have its risks. Because each person and each situation is so unique, what may work for somebody else may be ineffective or even dangerous for you. Here's where common sense, intuition, and your own personal experiences are vital in choosing strategies to heal yourself.

Learning from a book, even this book, has its limitations. Some of the concepts about healing and the strategies to make it happen that are described here may not work for you. This will not mean that you are abnormal or incurable (or that this is not a good book!); it may simply mean that you should seek out people with another set of experience. Talk to your grandmother or someone else's grandmother.

Everybody, indeed, has their own experience. Everybody is a grandmother with her own recipe for health and good living. This isn't to say that every recipe will work for you or that it even always worked for your grandmother. But if you think about it, your grandmother made it to her ripe old age doing something right. When everything else fails, try to emulate success.

20

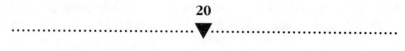

OBSESSION WITH HEALTH CAN MAKE YOU SICK

A halo only has to fall a couple of inches to become a noose.
Farmer's Almanac

If there were an organization called Healthaholics Anonymous, it would, no doubt, be immensely popular. Growing numbers of people are becoming more than just concerned about their health; they are becoming obsessed with it. These people are not simply interested in exploring specific health strategies; they are *into* them. They are into macrobiotics, into massage, or into yoga. Such people can become macroneurotic, or needy kneaders, or get so far into their yogic positions that they can't get out of them.

There is a real difference between concern about health and obsession with it. People obsessed with nutrition believe that there are only two types of foods: those that are good for you and those that cause slow, painful death. People obsessed with stress-management strategies spend so much energy managing their life that they neglect to live it. People obsessed with taking vitamins turn useful supplements into potentially dangerous substances. And people obsessed with meditating may end up sitting on all their other needs.

The most common obsession in the health area is with food. Anyone who starts to research the various theories about nutrition ultimately discovers that almost any food is thought to be poison according to at least one school of thought. Meat is poison to vegetarians, milk products are poison to vegans, tomatoes and eggplant are poisons to macrobiotics, cooked foods are poison to the raw foodists, and on and on.

For every reason someone might give that a food may be bad for you, someone else can give another reason why that same food provides certain benefits. Meat may have too much fat, but it is also often an excellent source of iron. Eggs may have cholesterol, but they have lecithin in them that helps digest cholesterol and other fats more effectively. Cooked foods may lose certain nutrients, but they make other nutrients more assimilable. Even ice cream can be an important "mental-health food."

For people obsessed with nutrition, perhaps the most dangerous thing they are ingesting is their own fear; fear of pesticides, hormones, fluoridation, chloridiation, radiation, and heavy metals is ingested with every meal. You can only wonder if their emotional state is poisoning them more than the food.

Obsession with exercise is also common. Although this obsession may seem more beneficial than harmful, the dark side of exercise fanaticism becomes evident when exercise begins to dominate your life. When you begin to live for the gym or your fifty miles a week, when your personal relationships begin to suffer because your exercise routine always comes first, when you exercise in spite of injury, or start climbing the walls when you can't work out, you may wake up one morning to discover that the only thing left in your life *is* exercise. And that's about as unhealthy as you can get. The purpose of good health and exercise is to enrich your life, not to *become* your life.

The exercise addiction is particularly problematic when you become obsessed solely with workouts and neglect other valuable ways to build and maintain health. The athlete who eats junk food and the bodybuilder who can't relax are two classic examples. Although there are certainly worse addictions than exercise, any action that limits your freedom diminishes your health.

One way to know if you are obsessed with health is if you realize that you are passionate about a single health discipline, be it nutrition, exercise, homeopathy, herbs, or yoga but ignore other strategies. Health is feeling whole; it should be a balance of the physical, emotional, mental, and spiritual aspects of our being.

It is certainly healthy to be concerned about your health, but obsessions and addictions fragment the wholeness of health and ultimately disrupt the quality of your life. As members of Healthaholics Anonymous might someday say, "May God grant me the serenity to accept the health conditions I cannot change, the courage to heal myself of the ones I can, and the wisdom to know the difference."

21

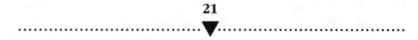

A POLLUTED PLANET CREATES POLLUTED PEOPLE

The creature that wins against its environment destroys itself.
Gregory Bateson

Our planet is not called Mother Earth for only symbolic reasons. We have been born of this Earth. We are not simply on this planet but *of* this planet. Unless we learn to take care of our home, we will all be prematurely buried six feet under it.

Just as the human body can become ill, so can a planet. Pollution is turning the Earth prematurely gray. Global warming is a fever, an inflammatory condition that is slowly cooking us all.

The life-giving blood of the planet is diseased with water pollution, and the planet's respiration is being choked by air pollution. Our planet's most efficient oxygen-manufacturing plants are the rain forests and they are being wiped out. Anemic soil conditions are creating biological malnourishment and chronic fatigue, turning lush plant life into desert. Overpopulation is creating congestion, a type of constipation of increased waste build-up with diminished capabilities of elimination. Toxic waste sites have become the planet's newest infections; corrosive sores oozing and seeping out wherever they can. And the greatest long-term potential danger to our Mother Earth is nuclear waste storage, which creates a hereditary disturbance that can strike at the heart of the planet's life. Such storage becomes the Earth's legacy. It is a Pandora's Box that must never be opened, yet we can only *hope* that time and circumstance do not disturb it.

Like the human body's response to symptoms, the planet's symptoms are its efforts to call attention to a problem, to reduce the effects, and to heal itself. Sometimes, however, the stress is overwhelming, and the Earth cannot heal itself adequately or rapidly enough against the ravages of the human race. It adapts; it deforms itself, and it rids itself of any vulnerable life form— even if that means destroying its children to save itself.

Efforts to control, outwit, or dominate nature are ultimately detrimental to human health and survival. Human health is more dependent on the health of the planet than the planet is dependent on human health. Unless we learn to live in harmony with our planet, we will be expelled from this once pristine Garden of Eden.

The 1990s are becoming the decade in which we are waking up to the need for a healthy home, both for our own benefit and for our planet's. More active efforts of conservation, recycling, and using biodegradable products are finally becoming planetarily patriotic.

There are innumerable decisions that each person makes every day that can slightly and sometimes greatly reduce the Earth's resources. We must make these decisions more consciously so that we learn to live in greater harmony with our home.

One of the most effective ways to help the Earth heal (and yourself too) is by becoming a vegetarian or at least eating less meat. Eating lower on the food chain is less energy intensive, less polluting, and more ecologically beneficial than our standard American diet. Not only must more people purchase recyclable products more often, we must also consume less. Not only must more people conserve energy, we must seek alternative forms, such as solar and wind energy. There are numerous books available that provide more suggestions for how you can help heal the Earth in your daily life.

Not only must we try to reduce the trouble that our lifestyle creates for our environment, we must also encourage the companies for which we work and the companies with which we do business to become ecologically concerned, both in the products they create and how they manufacture them. Ultimately, every action and every purchase must be considered for its environmental effect.

Although these efforts are vital for our survival and that of our children, we must still do more. Due to the already present environmental problems, we must now go on a planetary diet. We must extend our efforts beyond simply maintaining the Earth as it is to ways that will help the Earth recover from her severe illness. It is incumbent upon us all to strongly encourage governments to make more forthright efforts to clean up the mess we have created.

It has been said that one person's right to wave a fist ends where another's nose begins. Because everything on this planet is so interconnected, its nose, metaphorically speaking, is actually much larger than most of us realize, not just to fists but to every kind of environmental assault. Each one of our actions has repercussive and cascading effects. Unless we learn to live lightly on our planet, our children will carry the heavy burden of our conscious and unconscious indiscretions.

▼

22

LOVE IS NATURE'S PSYCHOTHERAPY

*Love cures people—both the ones who give it
and the ones who receive it.*
Karl Menninger, M.D.

Everything is contagious; not just germs, but good vibes and bad vibes too. Witness what happens when a person begins laughing hysterically; see how soon this gets others to laugh or at least smile. Witness also what happens when someone is expressing hatred, and notice how other people around tighten their bodies, develop defensive postures, or maybe clutch someone's hand.

Loving and hating are not merely emotional states—both have direct physical effects on the body. Just as fear creates the fight or flight reaction, feelings of hate create an armoring of the body that tenses the muscles, raises blood pressure, shortens and speeds respiration, and creates a clear psychological distance between people. Feelings of love, in contrast, reduce tension, decrease blood pressure, lengthen and slow breathing, and blur the distinctions between one person and another. Not only does hate hurt others, it hurts the person feeling it, while love benefits both the giver and receiver.

Although most people do not know how to tell their body to heal itself, they do know how to love, and this can set the wheels of healing in motion. As Yale surgeon Bernie Siegel states, "If I told patients to raise their blood levels of immune globulins or killer T-cells, no one would know how. But if I can teach them to love themselves and others fully, the same changes happen automatically. The truth is: Love heals."

Love can heal physical, emotional, and spiritual pain. Love of self and love from or for others can soothe physical pain, enrich emotional life, and help connect you with others. Although love has powerful side effects, they are all positive. And when love doesn't heal completely, it at least makes the pain a lot easier to handle.

Learning to love is, however, a lot more difficult than it seems, especially for people who haven't received much love themselves. It is also difficult for those who have received what was *called* love from parents who tended to smother rather than soothe them. Perhaps the best place to start is by learning to love yourself. In the words of the Beatles song: "The love you take is equal to the love you make." By being loving, you make yourself more lovable. Through giving, you receive. By being joyful, you share joy with others. It seems so obvious, and yet it is so elusive to too many of us.

"As you sow, so shall you reap" is an old saying that reminds us that what we put into something is what we get back. The hands that give away flowers retain the fragrance of the gift.

Bad vibes can be just as contagious as good ones. Anger, fear, and hate are all contagious too, though each of us can learn to be more resistant to these infections. By expressing compassion, anger is dissipated. By seeking to understand the unknown, fear disappears. By loving, hate evaporates.

The price you pay for hating others is loving yourself less. Even worse, the body feels this emotion and expresses it as pain and disease.

Perhaps one day soon more doctors will prescribe love for their patients. It may not cure them all, but it is a wonderful place to start.

Part II

The One-Minute
(or so)
Healing Strategies

INTRODUCTION

The previous section's "Steps to Healing" are an important appetizer for understanding the art of healing. Now, you are ready for the meat and potatoes (or the tofu and tomatoes) of this book.

Many of you probably rushed to this section before reading the first one. What's the hurry? Lily Tomlin once said, "For fast relief, slow down." Although it's normal to want to make your body stop hurting as quick as we can, it is important, sometimes even necessary, to *understand* healing in order to make it happen most effectively. This is not meant to make you feel guilty if you jumped to this section right away; it is simply to say that the first part of this book contains important information that will make the following specific healing strategies work better for you. (Now's you're chance to go back if you missed it!)

Franz Kafka once wrote, "To write prescriptions is easy, but to come to an understanding with people is hard." Likewise, to take a vitamin, herb, or homeopathic medicine is easy, but to come to a real understanding of what is wrong with you and what you can do on a deeper level to make it right is more difficult. The first section of this book has provided some groundwork. Now the simple strategies for healing specific ailments laid out in this section will take you the rest of the way.

Between ten and twenty-five strategies are offered for each condition. You are not expected, or even encouraged, to use all of them to heal your ailment (see step 20: "Obsession with Health Can Make You Sick"). Try using a few of them one day and a few more the next day, until you discover the ones that are most effective for you.

The one-minute strategies derive from both Eastern and Western cultures, and from ancient and modern traditions. Some strategies are part of folk medicine, some are a part of the cutting edge of contemporary medicine, and some will become an integral part of twenty-first century medicine.

Using unconventional methods

Some of the strategies recommended in this book are presently considered by the medical establishment to be unconventional or unproven. And yet, many of them have been used for a considerably longer time than modern medical treatments; some indeed for thousands of years. The term *unconventional* also depends on where you are in the world. In many places the use of herbs has always been considered completely conventional. In the Far East, acupuncture and acupressure are totally accepted while our conventional medicine, including Cesarean-section births and artificial hearts, are not.

What is considered unconventional therapy today may be mainstream tomorrow, and what is considered conventional medicine today may be tomorrow's quackery. This isn't a prediction; this is the evolution of medicine and science. Ultimately, the words *medicine* and *science* should be thought of as verbs, not nouns, for they are always changing, growing, transforming.

Physicians too often overestimate the risks and underestimate the value of using unconventional therapies. At the same time, they tend to overestimate the value and underestimate the risks of conventional therapies. A healthy scientific attitude toward these presently-unaccepted treatments is to maintain an open mind (but not such an open mind that your brain falls out).

On the other hand, it is important to seek conventional medical care when appropriate. If you have a potentially serious problem or recurring symptoms that are not remedied by the strategies recommended in this book, you should seek out professional medical care.

Ultimately, a collaborative approach that integrates natural and conventional treatments for healing may be the best way to make it happen.

Using this part of the book

This part of the book provides specific strategies to help heal yourself. Just as doctors practice medicine, you have to practice healing yourself. It is often necessary to experiment with one healing strategy or another—or a group of strategies. Such is the adventure of practicing healing and practicing life.

Although some people who have never tried, or rarely used, natural therapies may feel uncomfortable with them, it is reassuring to know that natural healing strategies are generally safer and have been used for a considerably longer period of time than conventional medical treatments.

Have fun with these remedies. Learning to utilize herbs with all their unusual textures and pungent fragrances is an enjoyable and empowering experience; pretend that you're a primitive medicine woman using herbal wisdom that has been passed on for generations in your tribe, or a shaman learning the secret languages of body and soul. Discovering the immediate effectiveness (with no side effects!) of homeopathic medicines is very exciting, as is the detective work sometimes necessary to figure out the remedy to take for a particular set of symptoms. All of the strategies, from food choices to breathing exercises, will give you a sense of healthy control and connection to your body that is impossible to get from popping a laboratory-created pill.

This book is not intended to provide detailed information about every type of natural therapy. This book does provide an appendix in part 3 on the proper use of homeopathic medicines, which is important for you to read if you have never used them before. However, in order to fully enhance your understanding of *all* the recommended treatments and how to use them most effectively, I strongly urge you to educate yourself further by checking out the books in the recommended reading list at the end of this book.

Most of the suggested remedies are available at health food stores and at select pharmacies. To help you find local sources of these products, you may want to contact health practitioners in your area who specialize in natural healing. Because no health-food store or pharmacy stocks every supplement, herb, or homeopathic medicine, addresses for mail-order companies that specialize in these products are provided in Part 3.

You are now ready to embark on the adventure of using these

one-minute strategies for health and healing. Enjoy the process and, by the way, if you find that some of the strategies are taking longer than sixty seconds (it just might happen!), just put your stopwatch away, relax, and realize that your inner doctor has more patience than you know.

ACNE

▼

Acne is an all-too-common problem for teenagers, but is experienced by many adults as well. It is one of those conditions that isn't painful or even physically discomforting, however, it certainly is a blow to the ego. Acne can turn a pretty face into a

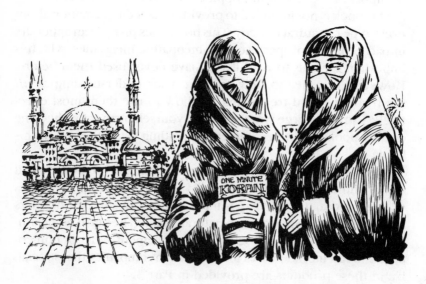

Acne is not a serious problem for Muslim teenage girls.

battlefield where bombs have exploded, soldiers are bleeding, and no side is winning. It is easy to feel that acne is nature's revenge against the beauty of adolescence. The good news is that you'll grow out of acne ... usually.

For those adults who haven't, it can be even more embarrassing than it is to adolescents. (The silver lining here is that people may think that you're a teenager.)

On a more serious side, it is important to realize that skin symptoms are not necessarily a skin disease. Skin symptoms usually are signs of an internal problem manifesting itself on the skin. The skin is considered the third kidney—it is another organ of elimination that the body uses to externalize oils and other matter not excreted from the body in the urine or stool. Because acne is as much an internal problem as an external condition, it is not enough simply to wash your face regularly. Treating skin problems is also an inside job.

Having acne isn't all bad. Who knows? Texture may be in next year. If, however, this isn't your idea of a fashion statement, try these strategies.

Clean up your act

Hygiene is important, and you can benefit from washing your face two or three times a day. If you use make-up, make certain to wash it off every night.

Too clean is too much

Avoid using soaps that dry out the skin or cause redness. Avoid using alcohol as an astringent because it tends to dry out your skin too much. Witch hazel solutions are more effective astringents.

An herbal wash

Take tincture of myrrh, dilute it in a small bowl of water, and use a swab of cotton to wipe your face. Myrrh's antiseptic and astringent properties can both treat and prevent acne.

Oil's well does not always end well

Avoid oil-based cosmetics because they tend to clog skin pores. Cosmetic-induced acne is a common problem for many women. Look for cosmetics labeled "non-comedogenic."

Your hair is contagious

Your hair secretes oil. Keep it off your face with a comb or brush. Wash your hair at least every second or third day.

To squeeze or not to squeeze

Most pimples should not be squeezed; a pimple is an inflammation, and you can cause infection by breaking it open. In particular, whiteheads should not be squeezed. On the other hand, you can speed the healing of blackheads and pimples with yellow pus by gently squeezing them. It is best to apply a clean, hot, wet cloth or tissue to help soften the pimple, allowing you to break it open with gentle pressure. Make certain that your hands are clean when you do this.

Supplement yourself

Vitamin A, vitamin B-complex, vitamin E, and zinc are helpful supplements for treating acne. Vitamin A can be used in an ointment, cream, or pill. Treatment with 135 mg. of zinc was found to be at least as effective in treating acne as antibiotics such as tetracyline—and without its potentially serious side effects (this high dose of zinc, however, should be used only under medical supervision). Some experts suggest zinc picolenate or effervescent zinc sulphate as the preferred forms for acne treatment.

Garbage inside, garbage outside

Acne can be affected by the food you eat. Although no foods have been proven to cause acne in all sufferers, some people have adverse reactions to milk products, nuts, fats, fried and oily foods, and chocolate.

Emotional garbage inside, emotional garbage outside

Emotions may be eating at you, literally. Emotional turmoil can disturb digestive and endocrine functions, leading to inefficient digestion of oils and a potential increase in skin oils. The first step to deal with any emotional problem is to acknowledge it. Don't deny your emotions, but don't let them get the best of you either. Next, express what you are feeling; don't suppress it, or you may next experience it on your face.

Face relaxation

Research has shown that people with acne have higher levels of anxiety and anger than others. However, this research didn't discover if the anxiety and anger lead to the acne or if the acne leads to anxiety and anger. In any case, it is worthwhile to do something so that these emotions don't take a more serious toll on your health (or on your face). Relaxation exercises may help you lessen your anxieties. Consider meditation, progressive relaxation, breathing exercises, or yoga.

There is a difference between cosmic beauty and cosmetic beauty

Everyone has their own inner beauty. Once you truly recognize this, you'll reflect it, and become even more beautiful.

ALLERGIES
....▼..

These strategies primarily focus on the treatment of allergies with respiratory symptoms. If you have other symptoms of allergy, such as asthma, constipation, ear infections, fatigue, diarrhea, headache, indigestion, or nausea, see the appropriate section.

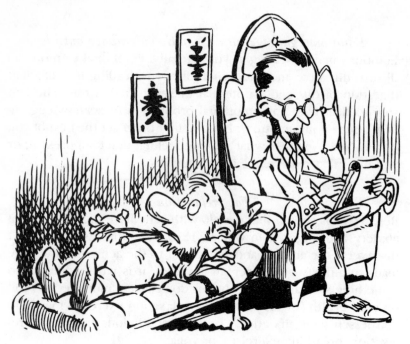

*Sneezy has had a serious identity crisis
ever since his allergies were cured.*

Freedom from allergies is nothing to sneeze at. This freedom, however, is a distant dream for many allergy sufferers.

Allergies can be imprisoning. They can make it impossible to go for a walk in the country, and even make it difficult to go outside at all. Some allergy sufferers can't visit their friends who have pets, and many others can't eat their favorite foods.

Even the pleasures and benefits of exercise are difficult because some allergy sufferers' noses run more than they do. A runny or stuffy nose leads to mouth-breathing, then a dry mouth, then less-efficient breathing, and then less-efficient overall functioning. A domino effect is set up, and the allergy sufferer is knocked down.

Conventional medical treatment for allergies usually consists of antihistamines, steroids, and desensitization shots. In obstinate cases, laser surgery may be utilized to vaporize mucus-forming nasal tissue. Be very careful of these treatments however, since they all have side effects. Worst of all, these treatments may be the prelude to the most serious of all allergy treatments: cutting off the nose. (Not really, I just wanted to shock you.)

Perhaps the greatest misunderstanding about allergies is the assumption that the allergen (the cat dander, the pollen, the housedust mite, or whatever) is the problem. Actually, the allergen is simply the trigger, while the allergic person's body is the loaded gun. Rather than just treating symptoms, or avoiding the allergen, the best course is to take action to strengthen the body's own immune and defense system. Natural therapies which do this help empty the loaded gun or simply make it shoot blanks.

Unless you own stock in Kleenex and don't mind purchasing it in bulk quantities, consider the following strategies. Some of these will strengthen your body and potentially reduce your allergies, while others will primarily reduce your exposure to the allergen.

Be breastfed
This isn't really a one-minute strategy for you, but it can be an effective strategy for your infant. Breastfeeding reduces the risk of having allergies later in life.

Take a shower and wash your clothes more often
Your body or your clothes can carry the pollen, cat dander, or other substances to which you are allergic. You may be continually reinfecting yourself.

Wear natural-fiber clothing
This especially applies to natural undergarments. You may be allergic to certain synthetic fibers.

Wash your pillow
One of the most common sources of allergies is dust mites which can inhabit the inside and outside of a pillow. Although they will make their home in synthetic substances as easily as they will in

down or foam, synthetic pillows have the advantage of being washable.

Dry out
Use dehumidifiers and air conditioners to dry out a humid room. Molds and dust mites tend to grow in humid rooms.

Ventilate your car's air conditioner
If you plan to use your air conditioner, run it with the windows open for five minutes before getting into the car. Also, there are products available that decontaminate your air conditioner; try to do this once a year. You should also consider decontaminating your humidifer by flushing it with one-half cup of liquid bleach to a gallon of water, as often as once a week if you use it frequently.

Create a dust-free room
Those dust mites and molds can hide anywhere—in carpeting, drapes, and even in teddy bears. Vacuum frequently; don't neglect washing drapes, and keep away from stuffed animals unless they have been washed recently.

Get a pet alligator
Although many people with allergies are allergic to various kinds of animals, it is rare to be allergic to reptiles or fish. Consider getting a pet snake, lizard, or fish. This won't necessarily cure your allergy, but it will give you a friend to love, which may be at least somewhat therapeutic.

Don't drink and sneeze
Alcohol can aggravate an allergy because it causes swelling of the mucous membranes. So don't drink and sneeze; you may blow yourself away.

Put the pressure on
Acupressure points all along the cheek bones and at the base of the nostrils help open the sinuses to clear your nose. Use your

thumbs to apply pressure for three to five seconds; let up, and then reapply the pressure.

Eat your honey

To be more precise, eat your local honey. There are very small doses of pollen in honey which sometimes can help immunize the allergy sufferer to the pollen. There are also various pollen products on the market, though the best results will come from pollen grown close to home.

Vitamins to blow your allergies away

Take 1,000 mg of vitamin C three times a day and 400 IUs of vitamin E twice a day.

Sting those allergies

Research has found that the freeze-dried herb stinging nettle (*Urtica dioica*), has significant effects on upper respiratory allergy symptoms. Freeze-dried preparations of stinging nettle are available in capsule form in quality health-food and herb stores. (I wouldn't recommend applying fresh stinging nettle directly to the nose. Use the freeze-dried; it's a little easier on it.)

Skunk cabbage is a great remedy for hayfever

Make tea of this herb, and drink a cup at least twice a day.

Miso your allergies

Miso soup, which is made from fermented, aged soybean puree, contains enzymes that aid digestion and can relieve symptoms of allergy.

Milk is not for every body, despite what the ads say

More people are allergic to milk and milk products than to any other food. Nature made cow's milk for calves, not humans. Avoid it as much as humanly possible.

Pollinate yourself homepathically

If you have hayfever, you can temporarily alleviate your symptoms with a combination of homeopathic medicines made from common flowers. Research published in the *Lancet* showed this to be a very effective treatment. Various homeopathic companies have allergy and hayfever products that contain common pollens. Take this medicine every four hours while you have symptoms, and stop once the symptoms have dissipated. If you don't notice results within forty-eight hours, seek a more individualized homeopathic medicine after looking in a homeopathic guidebook (or try another strategy).

Make peace with whatever you are allergic to

Just because you are allergic to cats doesn't mean that you have to hate them. You can still appreciate these wonderful creatures—at a distance. This may not rid you of your allergy or even your symptoms, but it certainly feels better than cursing the cat, the pollen, or the molds.

ANEMIA

▼

People with anemia may have the blahs, or, in the language of television, have "iron-poor blood." Besides being easily fatigued, people with anemia often have pale complexions (eeeks!), dizziness (whoops!), headaches (ow!), brittle nails (oh my God!) and even depression (ohhhhhh noooooo!). But yes, anemia-sufferers—there is hope.

Anemia is a reduction of the oxygen-carrying capacity of the blood. It is a type of suffocation that the blood experiences because of inadequate nutrition, a loss of blood due to injury or disease, or certain diseases—such as sickle cell anemia—in which the body's red blood cells are being destroyed.

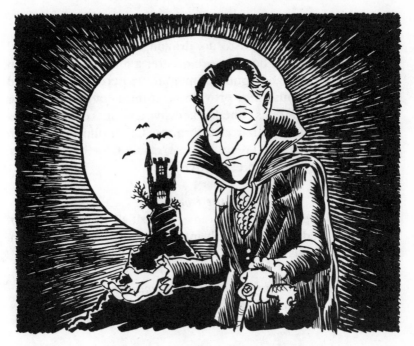

Anemic people create lethargic vampires.

Those more likely to have anemia are those who have increased iron needs: women, because they menstruate; pregnant and lactating women, because of their increased nutritional requirements; people with gastrointestinal disorders, because internal bleeding leads to blood loss; strict vegetarians who do not eat any meat or dairy products; aspirin-users, because this drug can cause internal bleeding; children, who are in a growth phase; and the elderly, due to poor iron absorption.

Anemia isn't a disease; it's a symptom of disease. It is a sign and signal that the body isn't able to oxygenate its blood adequately. The following strategies are relatively easy. However, if your condition does not improve within a couple of weeks, consider medical care. In the meantime, avoid vampires. Additional loss of blood may aggravate your condition.

Pass on the coffee, tea, and soda

Here are some things *not* to do: drinking coffee, black tea, and sodas, especially one hour before or after a meal, since they can interfere with iron absorption from 40 to 95 percent! Coffee and tea drain you because they provide short-term energy but create long-term fatigue. Sodas contain excessive amounts of phosphates which can interfere with iron absorption. Other phosphate laden products are beer, ice cream, cheese, candy bars, baked goods, and EDTA (a common preservative).

Avoid the iron Scuds

Chocolate, blueberries, and summer squash all contain a type of chemical called oxalate, which interferes with iron absorption. Avoid these foods that shoot iron down.

Eat red things that nourish your red blood

Eat liver (if organic), cherries and cherry juice, eggplant, raisins, prunes, and the seaweed dulse.

Pump iron

Other foods that contain a lot of iron are white chicken meat, dark turkey meat, blackstrap molasses, sunflower and pumpkin seeds, oysters, eggs, brewers yeast, and green leafy vegetables.

Take iron supplements . . . carefully

Because iron supplements can interfere with zinc absorption and destroy vitamin E stored in the body, this mineral should be taken with care. You shouldn't take a supplement larger than the recommended daily allowance, between 10 and 30 mg. (except under medical supervision).

Vitamins C and E promote iron absorption

Take 500 mg. of vitamin C twice a day, and 200 IU of vitamin E.

Beauty and the Bs
Proper amounts of folic acid and B_{12} are also important for absorption of iron. It is recommended to take 0.5 to 1 mg. of folic acid and 25 to 50 mcg. of B_{12} daily.

There's iron in them there herbs
Several herbs are rich in iron, and when made into a tea, they provide a healthy amount of iron. A combination of the following herbs is recommended: nettles, dandelion leaves, and comfrey. Nettle (also commonly called stinging nettle) is iron-rich. The dried (non-stinging) herb is readily available in health-food stores. Fresh nettles can be steamed and taste like spinach, but tastier. Just be very careful in handling them in their raw state, since their spines can cause a sharp, burning irritation.

Eat foods with copper in them
Copper helps the body assimilate the iron in foods. Foods which have copper in them are organ meats, seafood, nuts, legumes, molasses, and bonemeal (a supplement).

Expect to sink if you over-zinc
Over-consumption of zinc supplements can lead to copper deficiency, which can then cause anemia.

Don't overdo fiber or calcium
Fiber acts as a laxative, and too much of it can help wash iron out of your body before it gets absorbed. Also, some of the grains have (in their bran) a type of acid, called phytatic acid, which interferes with iron absorption. High calcium intake inhibits iron absorption, too.

ARTHRITIS

▼

Sir William Osler, considered to be the Father of Modern Medicine, once said, "When an arthritis patient walks in the front door, I feel like leaving by the back door." And it is no wonder that it pained Dr. Osler to treat the arthritic; there is little that conventional medicine can offer them. The lucky ones get temporary relief, along with drug side effects; the unlucky ones only get the side effects.

The term *arthritis* means inflammation of a joint, and there are various ways that people experience this. There are dozens of kinds of arthritis: osteoarthritis, rheumatoid arthritis, gout, systemic lupus, bursitis—to name just a few. The good news is that arthritis will rarely kill you. The bad news is that the stiffness

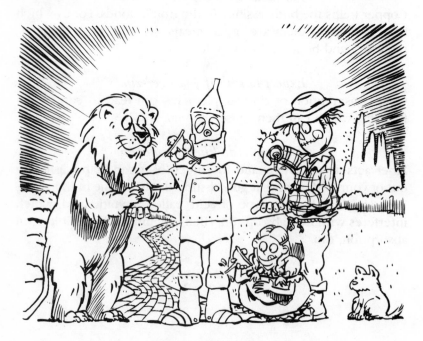

How arthritic stiffness is treated in the Land of Oz.

that you experience can make you feel like rigor mortis has set in early.

Osteoarthritis is the most common type of arthritis. Sometimes called the "wear and tear" variety of arthritis, osteoarthritis is thought to be a natural result of aging. This is just a theory, however, as demonstrated by the ninety-three-year-old man from Chicago who developed osteoarthritis in his left knee. When his doctor told him that it was a result of aging, the man remarked, "My other knee is ninety-three years old, too, and it don't hurt a bit."

There are other factors in addition to aging that precipitate osteoarthritis. Likewise, each type of arthritis has numerous influences that increase or decrease the chances of getting it. It is known, for instance, that women experience most types of arthritis two to eight times as often as men (gout and ankylosing spondylitis are the exceptions). Sorry, ladies, but sex-change operations are not therapeutically effective in this area.

Here, however, are some strategies that may help you.

Use it or lose it

Range-of-motion exercises are very important to increase circulation and reduce stiffness. Although one should avoid exercising a joint that is inflamed or "hot," these joints can be gently moved along their range of motion. Swimming is a particularly good exercise for people with arthritis. Although jogging is not associated with degenerative joint disease, you might consider walking instead if you experience any joint pain during or after jogging. Don't overdo any exercise, but don't underdo it either. Try to exercise fifteen to twenty minutes a day, five days a week.

Avoid arthritis cooperators

Some evidence suggests that certain foods can aggravate an arthritic condition. Although such foods are not thought to cause arthritis, they may make it worse. Avoid foods from the nightshade family, including tomatoes, eggplant, peppers (except black pepper), and potatoes (except for potato juice, discussed later). Tobacco is also a member of the nightshade family which can aggravate arthritis. Milk, citrus fruits, and fats are other known cooperators with arthritis and should be avoided or at least significantly reduced in your diet.

Cut yourself down to size
Avoid wearing high heels; they tend to place excessive pressure on certain joints and aggravate your condition. They can also hurt your posture.

Something to straighten you out and loosen you up
Researchers don't fully understand why, but sex, with or without a partner, has been found to relieve arthritis pain. Really.

Water yourself
Stimulate circulation in the affected areas by taking a hot shower or bath, then turning on the cold water. Repeat the hot cycle and then return to the cold. If your hands, knees, or feet are the primary sources of pain, you can place them in a tub or sink of hot and then cold water. Or put a hot pack on a specific area and alternate with a cold pack at least twice a day.

Become an opiate-like substance addict
Research has shown that the brain creates beta-endorphins—opiate-like substances that naturally reduce pain. Research has also discovered that there are lower amounts of beta-endorphins in the blood of some arthritis sufferers. Physical exercise and relaxation exercises both have been found to increase these natural painkillers.

A need for kneading
It doesn't take a rocket scientist to know that massage is good for arthritis. For the best results, avoid massaging directly on top of an inflamed joint. Instead, massage just above and below the joint.

Press a point near a joint

Press a pressure point that is near, but not on top of, the primary source of pain. You can find a good pressure point by feeling a slight crease in the skin (it will probably be tender). Press this point for three to five seconds, let up for a bit, then press it a couple more times in a similar manner. Some other good pressure points may be close to (not directly on) nearby joints. Try to press firmly but not too hard. Breathe into it; you will find that the pain lessens.

Cast castor oil on the pain

Make a castor oil pack and place it on a joint where there is pain—though not when there's acute inflammation. To make this poultice, pour three or four tablespoons of castor oil in a pan, heat until it simmers, then saturate a flannel cloth with the oil. After you place this cloth on the joint, cover it with a larger towel and place an electric heating pad over it. Keep it in place for thirty to sixty minutes.

Become a juice potato

An old folk remedy for arthritis is to drink raw potato juice. To make it, wash a potato (don't peel it), cut in into thin slices, place it in a glass of cold water, and leave it overnight. Drink this water in the morning on an empty stomach. The lowly potato is known to have antiviral inhibitors and is rich in chlorogenic acid, which helps prevent cell mutations that lead to cancer. Whatever it is in potatoes that helps arthritis sufferers is yet to be found, but personal experience suggests that it can be helpful.

Fish oil can lubricate you

Research has shown that fish-oil supplements have antiinflammatory effects that may be helpful for arthritis sufferers. One important study showed beneficial effects when people took fifteen capsules a day, though other research has shown that benefits can be expected from taking four to eight capsules a day. Recent research has also suggested that extracts from New Zealand green lipped mussels—now available in supplement form —are particularly good for people with osteoarthritis and rheumatoid arthritis. Although this supplement may sound strange, would you rather suffer or try something that may make you feel better?

Life should be a bowl of cherries

Some people report relief from arthritis symptoms after eating lots of cherries, especially in the treatment of gout. People with rheumatoid arthritis, or those who take aspirin frequently, may benefit from taking 500 mg. of vitamin C per day because they tend to be deficient in it.

Let herbs help you bend in the wind

Make an herbal tea with equal parts of alfalfa, chickweed, and yucca. You might also try using a Chinese herb called thundergod vine (*Tripterygium wilfordii*), which recent research has suggested is an effective treatment.

Bejewel yourself in copper

Some arthritis sufferers have been known to experience relief when they wear a copper bracelet. Although skeptics point to this treatment as a classic example of quackery, it is known that some people with arthritis have difficulty assimilating copper from the food they eat. Perhaps wearing a copper bracelet provides them with an additional source of this mineral. Lending further support to the use of copper, homeopathic physicians commonly prescribe microdoses of copper (*Cuprum metalicum*) to people with arthritis who experience cramping pains in the joints and jerking or twitching of muscles.

Sting arthritis pain

It is a well-known bit of folklore that beekeepers have a low incidence of arthritis. It is also known that one folk remedy for treating arthritis is getting stung by a bee. An easier way to try this remedy is to get a homeopathic dose of bee venom in *Apis mellifica 6* or *30*. This medicine is primarily helpful if you have arthritic pain that is similar to the type of pain that bee venom causes: burning pain, aggravated by heat, alleviated by cold or cool applications.

Poison ivy treatment

Actually, yes, but only homeopathic doses of it. Poison ivy, known as *Rhus tox* in homeopathy, is a very effective medicine if you have the "rusty gate" type of arthritis, that is, pain that is worse upon initial motion and reduced as you continue to move. If you have this pattern of symptoms, *Rhus tox 6* or *30* may be helpful to you. If, however, your pain is increasingly aggravated by any type of motion and is not alleviated by continued motion, take *Bryonia 6* or *30*.

Are you too resistant to change?

Is the stiffness in your character creating a stiffness in your body? There's the story of two caterpillers who look up and notice a butterfly. One caterpiller says to the other: "You'll never get me up in one of those." Are you resisting an inevitable change in your life? Loosen up. Say to yourself: "I expect change, and I will bend with this change."

ASTHMA

▼

Some people say that the best treatment for people with asthma is parent-ectomy. Although parental smothering can certainly be an influence, there are other factors that predispose people to both breathlessness and asthma.

Asthma is primarily an allergic condition, triggered by various

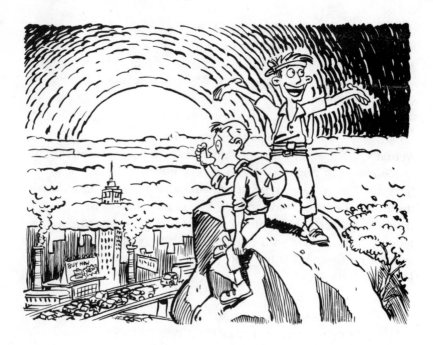

"Doesn't this view take your breath away?"

foods, preservatives, pollens, weeds, grasses, chemicals, fumes, the house dust mite, or tobacco. Emotional stress and vigorous exercise can also trigger an attack. If you find that something "takes your breath away," consider these strategies.

Just don't sit there, sit *there*

Relax. Feeling tense and anxious makes breathing more difficult. Being tense is like trying to untie a knot by pulling at both ends. Relax, and the knot almost unties itself. Progressive relaxation in which you first tense and then relax muscle groups is an effective way to achieve a heightened state of relaxation. Make sure to relax your shoulders; it's hard to breathe fully when your shoulders are up around your ears. (It makes hearing more difficult, too.)

Don't just sit there, move!

Certain exercises that strengthen the lungs can be very helpful. Swimming is best, especially the breast stroke. Aerobic dancing has also been found to help asthmatics. Start all exercise programs slowly, take rests when you feel a need for them, and don't overdo it. There were five gold medalists in the 1972 Olympics who suffered from asthma, so don't assume that asthma has to limit your ability to exercise.

Vacuum therapy

Perhaps the most common substance that triggers asthmatic breathing is the feces of the housedust mite. Vacuum as much as possible. Also, when you vacuum vigorously it can become an aerobic exercise, which in itself is therapeutic.

Give your skin the brush-off

Your skin is a third lung—it breathes and oxygenates you. Avoid covering your body with oil when you have respiratory problems, since you want to keep your third lung breathing freely. Take a louffa or any soft bristle brush and stimulate your skin.

Be cool

This one is easy: Turn the heat down. Many asthmatics have difficulty breathing in a heated room. Open a window too— unless you're chilled by it. Avoid too-cold temperatures; extremes of temperature can aggravate symptoms.

Humidify yourself

Humidifiers can help loosen the mucus that is blocking your breathing. You can potentiate the action of the humidifier by placing a teaspoon of eucalyptus, mullein, or thyme in a cold-mist humidifier or vaporizer. Make sure to wash the humidifier after each use. If you don't have a humidifier, put the oil into a pot of steaming water and place your face over the pot while you cover your head with a towel. Do this for as long as it feels good.

Preserve yourself; avoid preservatives

Certain preservatives, particularly sulfites and MSG, can trigger an asthma attack. Sulfites are often put in wine, beer, dried fruit, and seafood. They are also used in salad bars to keep the vegetables looking fresh. MSG is a common ingredient in Chinese food—ask the waiter or waitress to have your food prepared without it.

Breathergizing #1

Diaphragmatic breathing exercises your lungs and abdomen, and helps give you a full breath. To make certain that you're doing it correctly, follow these instructions. Place your hands on your waist above the hips. Your fingers should extend slightly over the sides of your lower abdomen, and the thumb should extend slightly over the sides of your back. Focus your attention on how your hands move when you breathe. Proper diaphragmatic breathing occurs when your hands are thrust out to each side, rather than thrust forward.

Breathergizing #2

Practice expiratory breathing. This is when you inhale normally, but exert slightly additional pressure during exhalation. Don't push too hard. This kind of breathing helps to dilate the bronchial passages. Do whatever visualization practices will augment this breathing exercise. For instance, imagine yourself pushing out the walls of a room. This may then give you more room for breathing.

Breathergizing #3

Take a full breath through your nose. When you exhale, pronounce, out loud, the syllables "woo," "ee," and "ah," on separate exhalations. Pronounce each syllable for five or six seconds. Gradually increase the length of your exhalations. After doing each syllable at least twice, you should be taking deeper, fuller breaths.

Bolster your breathing

Lie on the floor and place a bolster or large pillow under your upper back, just below the shoulders—your head should touch the floor. Slowly place your arms above your head; your chest will be lifted, and your back will be arched. Breathe fully into your chest and abdomen. Maintain this position for one to five minutes, but don't overstrain.

Do the cobra

The cobra is a yoga posture which aids asthma sufferers by opening their breathing passages. You begin by lying on your abdomen and placing your hands palms down under your shoulders. While inhaling and using your hands to support you, raise your head, then your chest using your back muscles. Try to raise yourself near the point at which your arms are straight. Hold this position, then exhale, slowly relaxing yourself back to the floor. Repeat this exercise at least five times.

Your lungs are in your hands

There is an acupressure point in your hands that will provide healing energy to the lungs. It is in the web of your hands between the thumb and index finger. You may notice that this area is very sensitive to pressure; this a sign that it needs to be pressed. Do so for at least five seconds and repeat it several times. Another good acupressure point to improve lung function is the web between your big toe and your second toe.

Supplement your breathing

Research has shown that 100 mg. of vitamin B_6 is helpful to people with asthma. You might also want to supplement this supplement with 1,000 mg. of vitamin C and 1 to 4 mcg. of B_{12} (the latter is especially good for sulfite-sensitive people).

Put spice in your life
Various pungent foods and spices have bronchodilating effects which can relieve symptoms of allergy. Of specific value are onions, garlic, chili peppers, horseradish, and mustard.

It's coffee time
Coffee also has bronchodilating effects. Research has shown that two cups of brewed coffee can relieve symptoms of asthma in one or two hours for up to six hours. Although the medicinal use of coffee may seem surprising to those involved in natural health care, you must remember that coffee, like every other herb, can be therapeutic in one dose and poisonous in another. Don't use this strategy if you are sensitive to coffee's other effects.

Is it a drug or is it an herb?
Ephedrine is a very popular drug that was once commonly given to people with asthma. Although this drug improves breathing, it also has various side effects, including nervousness, insomnia, increased heart rate, and dizziness. Because of this, it is not as popular as it previously was. However, there is an herb called Ephedra or "Mormon Tea," which contains ephedrine in smaller, safer doses. By making a tea of Ephedra with a half ounce of the branches in one pint of water and drinking one or two cups of it daily, you can receive the benefits of ephedrine without the side effects.

No smothering allowed
We all sometimes feel crowded, either physically or psychologically. While this doesn't bother some people, it can truly suffocate others. As they say in California, "Encourage others to respect your space." In other words, kindly tell people to avoid crowding you, either physically or with their expectations. At the same time, you might explore those characteristics in yourself that seek approval from others, desire attention, and want to be smothered.

Emotions allowed
Many people with asthma notice that attacks may be triggered when they bottle up their emotions. Allow yourself to feel whatever emotions you experience. Accept them and express them. The more they are bottled up inside you, the more they explode internally. Suppression of emotions can be enough to take your breath away.

Avoid cockroaches and chocolate
People with asthma are often allergic to cockroaches. Keep your house very clean to discourage cockroaches. Also, did you know that the F.D.A. allows manufacturers to have up to 4 percent by weight of cockroach parts in chocolate? It is apparently very difficult to keep these insects out of the chocolate vats (can you blame them?), so a good way to avoid cockroaches is to avoid chocolate. Strange, but true!

BLADDER INFECTION (CYSTITIS)
▼

The length of a film should be directly related to the endurance of the human bladder.
Alfred Hitchcock

Bladder infections cause frequent, urgent, and painful urination. Although not usually a dangerous medical problem, any condition that actually causes pain by doing so should be considered somewhat serious—if not by the doctor, at least by the patient. Approximately half of all women get a bladder infection at least once in their life and one in four women experience repeated bladder infections. It's enough to really—uh, tick, that's it—tick you off.

Bladder infections are much more common in women than in men. One reason is that a woman's urethra—the tube connecting the bladder to the outside of the body—is only one-half inch long, and this opening is so close to the anus that infection from nearby bacteria is relatively easy.

However, only approximately 50 percent of bladder infections are the result of bacterial infection. Other factors that trigger a bladder infection include a candida (fungal) infection, or an allergic response to certain foods or drinks. Vigorous sex and perfumed soaps can also irritate the urethra and the bladder. (It's ironic that getting down and dirty or getting squeaky clean can both create problems.) Vibrations, either from riding a motorcycle or from using a vibrator, can also irritate the bladder.

Antibiotics are not helpful for treatment except in the case of bacterial infections. Because antibiotics can disrupt the balance of helpful vaginal bacteria, the inappropriate use of these drugs can cause a candida infection. Get a culture to see if you have a bacterial infection and, whether it is positive or negative, consider these strategies.

Drink up!
Drink lots of fluid, but avoid coffee, black tea, caffeinated sodas, and alcohol, which can all aggravate your bladder. Try to drink at least eight glasses of water a day.

Take acid
Drink two or three glasses of unsweetened cranberry juice a day. This juice acidifies your urine and burns those bacteria or fungi out of your body. Taking 500 mg. of vitamin C three times a day also acidifies your urine. Some women report irritation from citrus fruits and spicy foods; it's best to avoid them.

Clean up your act
Sit in a tub of warm or hot water for twenty minutes. Put a half-cup of white or apple-cider vinegar in the water. Don't use soap. Make certain to keep your legs spread in order to cleanse the genital area. Repeat this in two hours and again, twelve hours later.

84

Empty yourself

Try to empty the bladder as often as possible, at least every three or four hours during the day. Try to urinate just before having sex and especially immediately after.

Get cultured

Eat unsweetened yogurt or miso soup at least once a day. Yogurt and miso provide helpful bacterial cultures to your body—particularly important if you are taking antibiotics.

Not so sweet

Bacteria thrive on sweet blood. Avoid keeping your blood sugar high by not eating too many sweets.

Be careful of hot pants

Tight pants or underwear not made from natural fibers don't allow adequate breathing. Synthetic fibers create an environment more conducive to bladder infections. Use only 100 percent cotton.

Reduce the pressure

An ill-fitted diaphragm can press against the urethra and ultimately irritate the bladder. Wide-lipped diaphragms put less pressure on the urethra. Speaking of sex, make certain to have thorough foreplay before making love (*not* a one-minute strategy). The woman should be adequately lubricated before the man inserts his penis. Also, the man should avoid scented condoms, since they may irritate the vagina.

Don't wipe yourself out

When you urinate, you should wipe from front to back. Wiping from back to front can spread anal bacteria to the urethra.

Herbal soothers

The following herbs should be mixed together and made into a tea: marshmallow (not marshmallows!), barberry (not blueberry!)

sage (not just any wise herb!) and horsetail (not on the type that will take you for a ride!). Mix them together and place approximately one tablespoon of mixture in a cup of boiling water; let simmer for five minutes and drink when cool. Drink one to three cups per day.

Animal wisdom

Cats and dogs eat couch grass when they have bladder problems. Couch grass has a high concentration of mucilage, which has a soothing effect on mucous membranes. Take one teaspoon of the root and simmer it for thirty minutes in one and a half pints of water. Drink cold, one swallow or one tablespoon at a time.

Spanish fly? Olé!

Spanish fly, commonly called by its Latin name *Cantharis* by those in homeopathic medicine, is very effective for certain types of bladder infections. If you have a great deal of burning during or after urination, frequent desire to urinate, and tend to pass urine only in drops, *Cantharis 6* or *30*, taken every four hours, should be tried. If it doesn't work within forty-eight hours, it wasn't the correct medicine and you can stop taking it. A different homeopathic medicine to consider is *Aconite 6* or *30* (monkshood) which is good for those bladder infections triggered by being chilled and which come on suddenly. When the bladder infection seems to be triggered by sexual intercourse, try *Staphysagria 30* (staveacre).

Clean up your act—carefully

Some women are sensitive to certain soaps, laundry detergents, bubble baths, contraceptive jellies, and dyes. Stick to natural, toxin-free products and avoid these potential irritants.

Speaking of emptying yourself

Are you pissed off and holding it in? Are you afraid to let go? Your body may be giving you a message. Remember, anyone can get angry, but to effectively express anger at the right person, at the right time, and in the right way is most therapeutic.

COLDS
▼

The common cold is the result of a viral infection, and mucus is a liquid vehicle that eliminates the dead viruses and the body's dead white blood cells that have valiantly fought the viruses. The nasal discharge that you experience with a cold is thus a healthy response to an infection.

Now that you know that this discharge is the body performing an important and healing function, you can understand that treat-

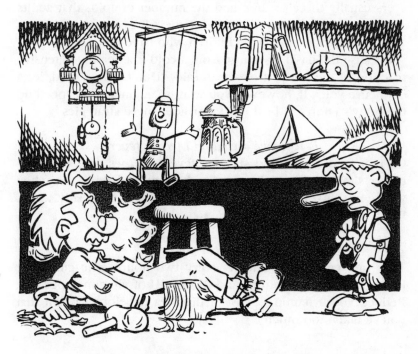

"I'm sorry, Gepetto. Next time I sneeze I'll use super-strength tissues."

ing it with a clothespin doesn't make sense. And yet, many people take over-the-counter cold remedies that have a similar effect. These drugs dry up the mucus that the body is creating in its effort to get rid of the dead viruses and white blood cells and heal the body. It is no wonder that such drugs only work temporarily and cause side effects, including congestion and drowsiness.

Scientists have identified over two hundred viruses that cause the common cold, and more are being discovered all the time. Despite our modern medical prowess, physicians and drug companies remain stymied on how to effectively prevent or treat this all-pervasive affliction.

The common cold lasts anywhere from two days to two weeks. Infants and children commonly get about six colds a year, teenagers usually three or four, and the number of colds that adults suffer tends to decline throughout their life, except for those adults who are exposed to children who have colds.

Because the nasal discharge from a cold is a healthy defensive reaction of the body, it has been said, "Don't cure a cold, let a cold cure you." If, however, you want to augment and speed up the body's efforts to heal itself, consider these strategies.

Is it starve a cold and feed a fever?

Or is it feed a cold and starve a fever? *Neither.* It is probably better simply to eat when you're hungry, and don't eat when you're not. Just make sure to get lots of fluids, especially water, broth, juices, and herb teas.

Supplement yourself

Take one gram of vitamin C every two hours, zinc gluconate lozenges every two hours, and 25,000 IU of vitamin A per day. Reduce your vitamin C dose if diarrhea develops (a sign that you've taken too much).

Get some fresh air

Because a cold impairs your breathing, it is important go outside, or keep windows in your house open (at least a little) in order to get fresh air and to optimize respiration.

Take a sauna

Sweat it out; it (the virus) may come out in the wash.

Don't get it handed to you

You are actually more likely to catch a cold from shaking the hand of a cold sufferer than by kissing. Cold sufferers shed their cold viruses onto their hands, then spread it to other people's hands, who eventually touch their nose or mouth and infect themselves.

Perhaps even more dangerous is nose-to-nose Eskimo kissing, although it may be therapeutic to the cold sufferer.

Let lemons squeeze the cold out of you

Lemons not only have vitamin C in them, they also have what one grandmother calls "natural corrosive action on mucus buildup." (One grandmother with a rather technical vocabulary, that is.) Make lemonade with equal parts of fresh lemon juice and water, add a pinch of cayenne pepper and some honey (not too much honey). This drink will work better when it is tart and hot. Don't boil the lemon juice; that will significantly reduce its vitamin C content. It is best to just heat the water first. Cayenne is known to help stimulate mucous membranes, loosen mucus, and increase circulation. Gargle with the first two gulps, and then drink the rest.

Herbal brews to bruise a cold

There are numerous herb teas that can help the body heal a cold. Brew one or more of the following herbs to make a tea: ginger (one ounce per pint of water), hyssop (one ounce per pint), peppermint (one-half ounce per pint), rosehips (one-half ounce per pint), and sage (one-fourth ounce per pint).

An herbal immune stimulant

Echinacea (purple coneflower) is one of the herbs that can pow-
erfully stimulate the immune system, helping it fight a cold more
effectively. At the first sign of a sniffle, cough, or sneeze, place a
dropperful (30 drops) of the echinacea extract in water. Drink
it once a day for three or four days.

Eucalyptus is a powerful natural antiseptic

One or two drops of eucalyptus oil in a bowl of hot water can
clear out your head quite rapidly. Put a towel over your head to
help trap the vapors, lean over the bowl, and inhale the eucalyptus
steam.

Garlic keeps the evil cold spirits away

Whether it's because garlic scares cold viruses or because the
enzymes within it devour the viruses, garlic can prevent the
development of a cold. It is most effective if taken during
the early stages of infection. Consider eating two to four peeled
raw cloves, (though you may want to consider this only if you're
staying away from people for the day). If you have to be around
others or you can't handle chewing on garlic cloves, there are
now odorless garlic capsules available that are equally effective.
Or try chewing on some fresh parsley afterwards. (It's a natural
breath-freshener.)

The old standby: chicken soup

Eat it as often as you think your mother would recommend it. It
really works!

No tears for onions

We all know that slicing onions can give us watery eyes and a
runny nose. Or more precisely, it causes a profuse, clear watery
and burning discharge that tends to irritate the nostrils. Because
they cause this pattern of symptoms, onions also can help to cure
them when given in homeopathic doses. Take *Allium cepa 6* or
30 (made from onions) every four hours if your symptoms match

this pattern. You won't need to take it for more than twenty-four hours.

Homeopathic vitamin C
Another homeopathic medicine to try is *Aconite 6* or *30* if your symptoms include a rapid onset of the cold after exposure to cold weather or a cold dry wind. Fever, restlessness, great thirst, and even a sense of anxiety may accompany the cold symptoms. *Aconite* is only effective if you use it within the first twenty-four hours after the symptoms begin. Take it every four hours. You won't need to take it for more than twenty-four hours.

Plant yourself
Indoor plants provide valuable moisture to the air and reduce the dry atmosphere caused by central heating, thus minimizing the drying effect on nasal passages and the throat.

Grow facial hair
Hair acts as a cold-virus filter when it's abundant around the nose and mouth. This strategy takes longer than one minute, it isn't appropriate for half of us, and it isn't fool-proof, but hey, anything that helps prevent a cold is welcome.

Run away from your cold
Research has shown that exercise temporarily stimulates white blood cells, thus helping fend off cold viruses. If, however, you're feeling achy or fatigued, don't exercise.

Drown your troubles in the ocean
If you live near unpolluted salt water and you're not chilled too much by swimming in it, go for a swim. Swimming in salt water stimulates your nose to drain ... and drain ... and drain....

CONSTIPATION

▼

*There is no disease but stagnation,
no remedy but circulation.*
Chinese proverb

When you realize that your large intestine is approximately five feet long and your small intestine is *twenty* feet long, it's amazing that anything finds its way out of your body at all.

So many people in Western society commonly experience constipation that many doctors dismiss it and consider it unworthy of their attention. Although constipation itself is not an illness, it is a symptom that something is wrong. Is your diet inadequate? Is there a stress in your life? Were you exposed to certain toxic substances? Is it a side effect from medication? Even though constipation won't kill you, it can lead to a general state of lowered health; sluggish stools lead to sluggish people, physically and mentally.

The most frequent cause of constipation is our processed, low-fiber, high-fat, and sugar-rich diet. Food companies have, for better and for worse, come to the aid of people with constipation and are adding fiber to everything. Ironically, to make white bread, food manufacturers commonly denature the whole wheat grain and then add fiber back into the bread. Some companies add powdered cellulose to their bread recipes. Although this certainly adds fiber to the diet, powdered cellulose—also known as sawdust—isn't the ideal way to get your fiber.

Older people are five times more likely to suffer from constipation than younger people. While this may be partly due to poor diet or lack of exercise, it is also connected to past laxative use. Millions of people today, especially the elderly, are addicted to laxatives. Although these drugs provide temporary relief, they do nothing to solve the cause of the constipation. Worse yet, whenever you get something done for you, eventually you won't be as able to do it yourself, leading to long-term constipation problems.

Most people don't realize that coffee has strong laxative properties. People sometimes become addicted to it, not simply for the taste or the caffeine, but because of coffee's effects on the bowels. People who sharply reduce their coffee intake tend to become constipated. There are safer ways to regulate your bowels.

Here are some strategies that you *can* do for yourself. They will be inevitably be helpful for navigating the twenty-five feet or more of intestines so that whatever you put into your body will be able to easily find the direction out.

Do, but don't overdo, fiber!

The best sources of fiber are grains, legumes, fresh fruits, and vegetables. Whole wheat bread and brown rice are naturally preferable to white bread and white rice. Bran, prunes, and apples are particularly good sources of fiber; however, be aware that increasing fiber intake too rapidly or simply eating too much of it can cause indigestion and diarrhea.

Lubricate yourself

Drink more water: a minimum of six glasses a day.

Bulk up

Take a bulk former such as psyllium preparations, available from herb stores or in commercial form from pharmacies (Try Metamucil or Konsyl. The latter is preferable because it does not contain sugar or NutraSweet). Flax or linseed are other good sources of bulk. At least once a day, grind some flax or linseed in a coffee grinder and add it to a cup of water, juice, broth, or cereal.

Olive oil and lemon

Take one tablespoon of olive oil and the juice of one lemon just before bedtime and first thing in the morning (don't eat anything for at least thirty minutes afterward). Commonly called a liver flush, this combination is thought to stimulate liver function and improve overall digestion and elimination of food. Another effective strategy is to mix the juice of one lemon with one cup of warm water and drink it before bedtime and upon waking.

Massage your abdomen from the outside and the inside

Massage your abdomen from the outside in a kneading-type of motion. Massaging your abdomen from the inside is another useful exercise: bend halfway over, placing your hands on your mid-thighs, exhale completely, and then empty your abdomen further by pumping your abdominal muscles up and down; try to do six pumps per breath. A more advanced internal massage is to pump the right side of the abdomen first, then the left side in the same breath.

Avoid laxatives, unless you want short-term relief and long-term constipation

If you feel you must take a laxative, take an herbal laxative, though the body can become reliant on herbal laxatives, too. Senna and cascara bark are probably the best. Place a teaspoon of senna leaves in boiling water and let them steep for thirty minutes. Drink a half cup in the morning and a half cup in the evening. Or take one tablespoon of cascara bark in capsule form before bedtime.

Avoid the drug plugs

If you are taking any medication, check to see if it causes constipation. Painkillers and antidepressants are two common types of drugs that usually cause constipation. Over-the-counter antacids that contain aluminum can also cause constipation.

Avoid the food and vitamin plugs, too

Certain foods, such as milk, cheese, and white-flour products, as well as certain supplements, such as iron and calcium supplements, can lead to constipation.

Exercise!
If your body is lazy, you can expect your stools to be lazy too.

Bounce in a squatting position
Flexing anal muscles by squatting and bouncing helps build anal muscle tone.

Get in touch with your inner plumber
When your intestines are not pushing things along like they should, perhaps a visualization exercise which imagines roto-rooter action moving things down the drain will help. This strategy may not be adequate if used without other strategies. Just like the Islamic saying, "Trust in God, but tie your camel," you should trust your inner plumber, but still eat your fiber.

COUGHS

It is common to feel uncomfortable when sitting close to a person with a cough. Not only is the sound distracting, a cough can expel air at a velocity of up to five hundred miles per hour. Such is the power of the body in its efforts to rid the respiratory system of irritants and toxins.

The cough is an effective primary defense of the human organism. It is therefore surprising that some over-the-counter drugs pride themselves on being a "cough suppressant." Besides being a questionable strategy in curing a cough, such drugs can delay the proper diagnosis of a serious illness such as lung cancer, emphysema, poisoning, or pneumonia.

The cough itself is not a disease; it is a symptom of a disease. Like other efforts that primarily try to control or suppress an individual symptom, drug treatments do not necessarily treat the underlying disease. A more healing therapy would be something

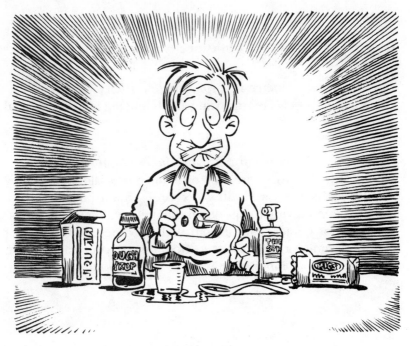

Another unproven treatment for the common cough.

that aids the body's efforts to clear respiratory obstruction or irritation.

There are innumerable types of coughs. There are dry and wet coughs, hacking and barking coughs, deep and shallow coughs, and single and rapid-fire coughs. Individualizing the treatment is important, though difficult. Basically, dry coughs should be treated first with humidification strategies and lozenges, while wet coughs can be helped by using natural expectorants. As for the various other types of coughs, you'll just have to experiment with different strategies, and don't forget to breathe. These strategies will point you in the right direction.

An expectoration cocktail
If you have a wet cough with mucus that obstructs your breathing, mix the juice of a lemon, one tablespoon of honey, and a quarter

teaspoon of cayenne pepper in warm water. The astringency and the acidity of the lemon causes the tissues to contract and helps to dissolve and dislodge mucus; the honey soothes the mucous membranes and respiratory tract; and the cayenne pepper adds power to the body's ability to expectorate. Gargle with this cocktail and then swallow it. Take as needed.

An expectoration cocktail for the brave
The onion is a great mucus-dissolver. Blend or juice an onion and add honey to it. Take a couple of tablespoons of this mixture as needed.

Other natural expectorants
Garlic! Eat a clove, if you're brave and not planning to entertain (or just take odorless garlic capsules). An easy strategy is making sage tea and adding garlic to it. Another herbal strategy is to mix elecampane and mullein. Elecampane is an herb which contains helenin, a powerful antiseptic and bactericidal alkaloid. Elecampane helps to expectorate the mucus, and mullein is soothing to the respiratory tract. For children, consider using wild cherry bark tea.

Treat your cough gingerly
Chew on a piece of ginger root and swallow the juice. Ginger has both anti-inflammatory and anti-oxidant agents which help to heal lung tissue and break up mucus congestion.

Herbal lozenges
White horehound is another herbal expectorant. White horehound lozenges are commonly sold in drug stores and health-food stores.

Vaporize yourself
Inhale steam from a vaporizer, or put a towel over your head and stand over the steam rising from a pot of boiling water. Consider adding a couple of drops of the herb hyssop to the water and

breathe this steamy air for five to ten minutes. Hyssop has been used since ancient times for its antiseptic and emollient (soothing) properties. Penicillin mold is known to thrive on its leaves.

Fire and ice treatment
Alternate hot and cold water in the shower, every three minutes or so. Make certain to get the water on your chest and your back.

Avoid milk products
The lactose in milk is a complex sugar that is difficult to digest for many people. It can encourage more mucus production, which further clogs breathing.

Where there's smoke, there's fire
Avoid first- and second-hand smoke. This irritant can exacerbate your breathing difficulties. If you have a cough and you're still smoking, remember that cancer cures smoking, permanently. Try a more agreeable cure.

Supplement your breathing
Vitamin C can help heal your cough if it is the result of a viral or bacterial infection. Take 1,000 mg. of vitamin C three times a day. Vitamin E can prevent and treat the cellular damage from cigarette smoke, dust, soot, pollen, smog, or other airborn pollutants. Take 400 IU of vitamin E twice a day.

Channel your mother
She is telling you to stand up straight so that you can take a full breath. She is also telling you not to wear clothing so tight that it inhibits your breathing. Now that you're thinking about your posture, do some exercises that will help it, such as stretching exercises that roll your shoulders back.

Relax your shoulders
Often you may find yourself walking around all day with tense shoulders. Shoulders should *not* normally be at or near ear height;

when you wear your shoulders as earrings, it is considerably more difficult to take a healthy deep breath. One good exercise to relax the shoulders is to lift them to your ears and tighten them, ... then relax.

Get loose
A cough tends to tighten your chest and back muscles, which then makes it more difficult to take a full breath. Do some yoga exercises that help you to loosen up a bit. Do the cobra: lie on your abdomen with your palms flat under your shoulders; lift your torso off the ground using your hands and arms, while keeping your head up and back; take several breaths in this raised position, and then slowly return to lying flat. Rest, then repeat this exercise several times. After this, do some back rolls: lie on your back and hug your knees as close to your chest as feels comfortable; gently rock forward and backward.

Chant your way to health
Unless speaking causes a coughing attack, try sitting in a relaxed position, making a single sound. It can be "ahhhhhhhh," or "ommmmmmmmm," or "yummmmmmmmm," or whatever feels good to you. Such sounds are soothing and can help to relax you so that the respiratory mucus falls into your digestive tract.

Keep the third lung healthy
Not only does your skin cover you, it also breathes for you. If you have respiratory problems, your skin often becomes more dry. Do not smear oily creams over it, which plug up the pores and make it difficult for this third lung to function. It's helpful to stimulate the skin with a louffa brush.

Re-spirit yourself
The very word *respiratory* contains the concept of "re-spirit." Are your spirits down? Have you noticed that you tend to breathe more shallowly whenever you're depressed? Such breathing invites a cough. Re-spirit yourself (see section on "Depression"),

and you'll find you'll take deeper breaths—then watch your cough spirit itself away.

DEPRESSION

▼

Depression is melancholy minus its charm.
Susan Sontag

Depression lowers your spirits and drowns you in sorrow, though tears aren't the only reason why when you're depressed you sometimes can't see straight. It caves in your chest, slumps your shoulders, and inhibits full breathing, usually forcing you to try to catch your breath by frequent sighing. You might say depression cuts you down to sighs. (My apologies.)

But depression is certainly more than physical. Its real ravages are psychological. It creates blah-itis, an inflamed state of the blahs. You lose interest in the things you normally love and begin really hating the things you weren't too sure about in the first place. You tend to doubt yourself and others; in fact, you doubt just about everything—except your own doubts. In more serious cases, you may wonder if life is meaningful or even worthwhile, and in the most extreme cases, you stop reading self-help books (pretty extreme, huh?). Hopefully, you haven't yet reached this terminal phase.

A major trauma can certainly be the cause that breaks you down, or you may get pushed over the edge by the accumulation of small stresses. You may feel depressed during what are usually thought of as good times, such as the holidays. Some women experience the baby blues shortly after giving birth. Every phase of life has its own potential for stress and depression.

But depression can also be precipitated by viral or bacterial infection, organic disease, or hormonal disorders. It can be drug-induced, especially from barbiturates, amphetamines, birth-control pills, or alcohol. It can stem from exposure to certain environmental poisons. It seems that sometimes depression can even be contagious; one person's low life condition can begin to bring others down with him.

With all these possible triggers floating around, it is no wonder that virtually everybody experiences some period of depression at least once in his life. There is no reason to feel guilty about an occasional bout of depression, unless, of course, you're trying hard to meet your annual guilt quota.

In every dark period in your life, there is also some light somewhere. Getting in touch with that light is important; in fact, it's just about the only way out. Of course, it's not always easy; it seems as though everyone has his own ideas about moving out of the depressed state of mind. Understanding the various theories about depression may be helpful in treating it, but remember what psychiatrist Carl Jung once said, "Learn your theories as well as you can, but put them aside when you touch the miracle of a living soul."

Whether you fully understand the reasons for your depression or not, here are some sensible strategies for reconnecting with and spreading your light.

Exercise those demons out of you!

Exercise is not only helpful for building a fit body, but it also helps to create a sound mind. Getting your body moving seems to help keep your mind out of the depths of depression. Exercise that involves the long muscles, such as jogging, swimming, bicycling, and playing basketball, football, or tennis, is the most beneficial.

Supplement your mood

A B-complex vitamin and the amino acid tryptophan are a good combination to take; they help increase the brain's release of serotonin, which is a natural anti-depressant. Foods that are high in tryptophan include bananas, soybeans, nuts, turkey, and tuna.

101

Don't overdo protein
Too much protein can inhibit the brain's intake of tryptophan and increase feelings of depression. Don't eat more than one protein-rich meal a day.

Don't forget to breathe
It is common for you to breathe shallowly when you're depressed, which tends to create a physical depression to go along with your mental one. You can help to get yourself out of this depressed state by taking full, deep breaths more often. Alternate-nostril breathing creates a rhythmic profusion of air, which further enhances oxygenation of the body. To do this type of breathing, sit comfortably with your back straight, exhale fully, close the right nostril with one finger and inhale slowly through your left nostril. After you have inhaled fully through your left nostril, close it and exhale through your right nostril. Keep your left nostril closed and inhale through your right nostril and so on. Repeat this process for a couple of minutes.

Befriend a friend
When you're depressed you tend to keep to yourself and wallow in your depression. Don't suffer alone—extend yourself; talk to someone or go visit a friend.

Help someone else
Being with, talking to, and helping others less fortunate than you will not only take your mind off your depression but will also help you feel better about yourself and your own life.

Befriend a pet
Having a pet cat, dog, tarantula, or whatever is wonderfully therapeutic. You have someone to talk to, someone who will listen to your every word, someone to provide you with unconditional love ... and a pet is cheaper than a therapist.

Give yourself credit for something

When you're depressed you tend to blame yourself for every-thing; you rarely acknowledge anything good about yourself or your life. Look for what *is* going right. By shining a little light onto the positive side, perhaps you will find that invincible sum-mer in your midst of winter.

Swear off sin

Alcohol, cigarettes, drugs (recreational *and* therapeutic) sugar, and junk food can all depress you, both physically and psycho-logically. Perhaps your depression is telling you that what you are doing to your body is bringing you down.

Join the coffee generation

Coffee, like sugar, can lead to various problems, but *small* amounts can also be beneficial for some people, especially during depression. Caffeine molecules have been shown to displace cer-tain neurotransmitters and help to keep the good-mood chemicals in circulation. Coffee is fast-acting and the effects can last three to six hours. Despite these benefits, though, be aware that coffee is like a drug; it has side effects. Because of this, safer methods should be considered before resorting to this strategy. Don't drink more than one cup per day during depressed times.

Let there be light

Light has been found to affect brain chemicals in a way that reduces depressive states. Try lifting the shades in your home, opening windows, turning on brighter lights, and wearing lighter and brighter clothing.

Get out of here

Consider travel therapy. Changing your routine, going on a va-cation, and adding a little adventure to your life is often thera-peutic.

Write on!
Keeping a journal of your thoughts, feelings, and experiences provides a wonderful catharsis. Writing can also help you come to a better understanding of your depression, which may help lift its veil so that you can better understand and appreciate yourself and your experience.

Draw it out of you
Draw or paint what you are feeling. Not only will it feel good to do this, you could create a valuable work of art.

Let it rain!
If the tears are there, cry! Don't bottle up your feelings. Tears contain chemicals that need to be released.

Say it with flowers
Yes, flowers often make a person feel appreciated but, in addition to giving or getting flowers, flowers can also be used therapeutically. The Bach Flower Remedies are thirty-eight flowers that British physician Edward Bach discovered to be beneficial for various emotional states. Dr. Bach found Sweet Chestnut, Mustard, and Crab Apple to be most useful for treating depression. These flower products are often available at health-food stores.

Pamper yourself
Give yourself time to appreciate yourself. Take a hot bath. Relax in a comfortable place. Listen to beautiful music. Get a massage. Take a walk in nature or any place that feels good to you. Read a good, uplifting book. Re-read this book!

DIARRHEA
....................................▼....................................

Diarrhea is, loosely speaking, the passage of too frequent, too soft stools. Diarrhea occurs when the fluid contents of the small intestine are so rapidly hurried through the large intestines that the fluid is not adequately absorbed and is then discharged.

Like vomiting, diarrhea is a defense that the body deploys in order to rapidly discharge germs, toxins, and irritants. Bacteria make up approximately 10 percent of the bulk of normal stools; this percentage increases if your diarrhea is due to eating bacteria-contaminated foods or drinks. Because of this high bacteria content, drugs that attempt to constipate someone with diarrhea can be harmful: they reduce the ability to discharge potentially dangerous germs. Often, it is best to let diarrhea run its course.

Diarrhea should not always be left untreated, however. Sometimes, diarrhea is symptomatic of a more serious disorder such as ulcerative colitis, which may require medical attention. And diarrhea can create its own problems, as in an infant whose diarrhea leads to dehydration. Still, the vast majority of people who experience diarrhea should not try to suppress this symptom immediately. Instead, here are some simple strategies that can help the body resolve itself.

Zen dieting
Eat nothing. Resting your digestive system often helps to reestablish healthy bowels.

Water yourself
Diarrhea leads to greater excretion of bodily fluids, so it is important to replace them by drinking lots of water. Persistent or acute diarrhea can also excrete important nutrients from the body. Since solid food is sometimes difficult to digest during bouts of diarrhea, drink diluted fruit juice with a pinch of salt. Alternate this with a glass of carbonated water that contains a quarter teaspoon of baking soda. Drink one cup after each bout of diarrhea. If fruit juice isn't available at the moment, try adding three level tablespoons of sugar and a half teaspoon of salt to a quart of water.

It's barbeque time, sort of

Take activated charcoal. This product is commonly sold in pharmacies and health food stores and has been found to stifle bacterial growth.

A pinch here and pinch there

Put a pinch of cinnamon and a pinch of cayenne pepper in two cups of boiling water, and let them simmer for twenty minutes. Take two tablespoons every hour.

Be good to your bowels, and they won't run out on you

Slippery elm bark is a tried-and-true herbal remedy for diarrhea—it's both nourishing and soothing to the bowels. Add one ounce of slippery elm bark to one quart of boiling water; let it simmer until approximately one pint remains. Add honey, if necessary, to sooth the palate, and take one teaspoon every thirty minutes.

Acupinch yourself

Pinch or press an acupressure point (Stomach 34), which is about two inches above the kneecap along the outside of the thigh. Another good point is Stomach 36, which can be found by placing the index finger and the thumb on either side of the kneecap. This places the middle finger on the correct point on the outside of the shin bone. If the spot feels a bit tender, you've found it. Press it for at least ten seconds, release, and then repeat a couple more times.

Eat the BRATY bunch

If you have an appetite, eat foods from the BRATY bunch: bananas, (white) rice, apple sauce, toast, and yogurt (not necessarily at the same time). These foods are nourishing and relatively easy to digest. Miso soup is also good.

Run to garlic

If you are diagnosed with parasites, eat lots of raw or capsulated garlic. (Parasites must not be Italian; they hate garlic.)

Arsenic, but not old lace
A homeopathic dose of arsenic (called *Arsenicum*) is an effective medicine for diarrhea caused by food poisoning. It can also be effective for diarrhea when you have what are considered the following *Arsenicum* symptoms: great thirst, but for only sips at a time; restless, but weak; chilly, but may also have a fever; and a worsening of symptoms at and after midnight. If your symptoms match the majority of these, take *Arsenicum 12* or *30* every four hours for one or two days.

Be anti-antacid and anti-antibiotic
Certain drugs create diarrhea as a side effect. Antacids have an ingredient in them that causes diarrhea, and antibiotics can kill beneficial bacteria, making it more difficult to absorb nutrients in the bowels, thus leading to diarrhea.

Don't drink just anything
Coffee, black tea, and alcohol can aggravate diarrhea.

Every body does not need milk
The American milk industry has tried to tell us that "Every body needs milk." This type of industrialized public-relations effort is messing with our minds ... and our bowels. Approximately 80 percent of black Americans, and 5 to 15 percent of white Americans are lactose intolerant. Milk is *not* good for every body—unless you consider running to the toilet to be good exercise.

Certain sugars aren't so sweet
Fructose and sorbitol (in sugarless gums and candies) can cause diarrhea. Avoid them if you have a tendency to this malady.

Avoid too much of a good thing
Fiber is good for preventing constipation, but too many fiber-rich foods, such as prunes, figs, and bran, can loosen you more than you may want.

Blame it on the bagels

Crohn's disease, a chronic diarrheal condition, is more often experienced by Jewish people than others. Unfortunately, converting to another religion will not be a very effective treatment.

Slow down

Do you talk fast, walk fast, drive fast, eat fast? Are you not finishing what you begin? Do you have a tendency to want to get something over with as soon as possible? Are you chronically running away from something? If you're not fully digesting your life and you always want to move on to the next thing before you're finished with what you're doing, your bowels may act the same way. Take your time. Don't hurry. Enjoy where you are. Repeat to yourself: I will learn to enjoy doing things slowly.

Anticipation is as strong as any bacteria

Anticipation can cause diarrhea just as effectively as bacteria can. Worries, anxieties, and other anticipatory emotional states can make your bowels feel insecure too. Repeat to yourself: I am at peace with myself and I appreciate where I am right now.

EARACHES
▼

Earaches are caused by many factors, including bacterial or viral infections, allergies, swimming, or changes in altitude from flying or mountain travel. Most commonly, earaches result when the eustachian tube, which connects the middle ear to the cavity behind the nose, is blocked, causing the trapped fluids to become a perfect breeding ground for bacterial or viral infection.

Doctors usually prescribe antibiotics for ear infections, however, these drugs do not always work. What's worse is that some research suggests that there is an increased probability of experiencing another ear infection when antibiotics are used. Sadly, too many doctors overprescribe antibiotics for earaches. Perhaps the medical community has its collective eustachian tube blocked so that it can't hear and respond to the research on the limitations of these drugs. When you realize that many earaches are caused by viral infection or allergies for which antibiotics are useless, it makes sense to seek out alternative treatment.

Because the eustachian tube in infants and children is sometimes too small or too short to work properly, they are more prone than adults to ear infection. In fact, earaches are the number one reason that parents take their child to a doctor.

Parents who are unfamiliar with a few simple home remedies inevitably feel helpless as they hear their child cry for help. In such instances, parents tend to feel more anxiety than the children feel pain. When the child gets recurrent ear infections, the parents' fear of potential hearing loss adds to the terror of the condition.

The following strategies are helpful for the little ears of children as well as those of the rest of us.

Treat a cold and sore throat well
If a child's cold or sore throat worsens, it can lead to an ear infection. Read the section on Colds and Sore throats so that you can help prevent ear problems.

Here's the rub
Massage the head, especially parts around the ear, though not the ear itself. Massage the parts that seem to feel sensitive to touch for at least a minute. Massage them for another minute after a short rest.

Be fluid
Earaches sometimes result from mucus congestion in the nose and throat. Be certain to drink enough fluids. Warm fluids tend to be more soothing. However, avoid drinking milk, which can lead to more congestion.

Whether you're tired or not, yawn
Yawning helps to open the eustachian tube, which can reduce ear pressure and help decrease fluid or pus build-up in the ear.

Chew your cud
Chewing and swallowing helps to open the eustachian tube, reduce ear pressure, and decrease ear pain. Try chewing some gum.

Steam it out
Steam inhalations or saunas may be helpful. These treatments create a pseudo-fever during which white blood cells become more active and can more effectively fight infection.

Avoid swimming
Being underwater can aggravate an ear infection.

Hunt for allergies
Some children are allergic to certain foods that weaken them and make them more susceptible to illness, including ear infections. Perhaps the most common culprit is milk and dairy foods. Every calf may need milk, but most humans don't.

Let garlic get the demons out of those ears
Peel a clove of garlic, dip it in oil, and place it at the ear's opening (do not push it into the ear). Leave it there overnight, unless it becomes too irritating.

Let's hear it for mullein oil
Place a couple drops of mullein oil into the ear. Mullein is an herb, and many pharmacies and most herb stores sell mullein oil. If there is discharge from the ear, it may indicate that the eardrum is broken. Do not use any type of ear drops if this happens.

For those little infant ears
Tincture of Plantago (plantain) is an excellent remedy for infants who are teething at the same time they are having ear pains. Make

the tincture by diluting two parts of the remedy to one part water. Place a couple of drops in the ear and rub some into the gum. This remedy is available at homeopathic pharmacies or herb stores.

Supplement yourself with culture

Because many people with ear infections have often been given dose after dose of antibiotics, it is important to help the body reestablish the healthy bacteria that ordinarily live in your intestines. Take an acidophilus supplement. The best strains are DDS and NCFM. (If a supplement doesn't say that it includes these strains, then it doesn't.)

It's as simple as ABC

There are three common homeopathic medicines for ear infection: *Aconitum* (monkshood), *Belladonna* (deadly nightshade), and *Chamomilla* (chamomile). *Aconitum* is usually given at the initial onset of ear symptoms, especially if it began after exposure to cold. *Belladonna* is given when a person with ear infection has a noticeably reddened ear, ear canal, eardrum, and sometimes a flushed face. There is a sudden onset of symptoms, with pains that are throbbing, piercing, or shooting, sometimes extending to the throat. These pains are worse by motion and night and better by sitting semi-erect and with warm applications. They usually have a fever concurrently. *Chamomilla* is indicated when the person, usually an infant, experiences great pain and is extremely irritable because of it. They are impatient and cannot be consoled. They are very sensitive to touch, though are temporarily relieved by being rocked or carried. They may experience teething concurrent with their ear infection. Take the 6th or 30th potency every four hours for one or two days.

A sure-fire cure for ear canal infection

If you get an earache because of water in your ear from swimming or showering, tip your head to one side, pull the top of the ear upward and backward to drain what water you can; then squeeze a dropperful of equal parts white vinegar and rubbing alcohol into the ear. The alcohol absorbs the water, while the vinegar kills the bacteria or fungi that are growing in your soggy ear. Although this is an old-time cure, it is now recommended by the American Academy of Otolaryngology (doctors of ear, nose, and throat).

Breastfeeding is the best feeding

Breastfed babies have been found to have fewer ear infections. Their immune system seems better able to resist infection, and they are less prone to allergies and the ear infections that sometimes result from them.

Correct your bottlefeeding and breastfeeding technique

Infants who are prone to ear infections should never be fed while they are lying flat. If they are lying flat, the milk has a tendency to go directly into the eustachian tube and block it, thus leading to ear infections.

Don't take your earache lying down

Most earaches in both adults and children are aggravated by lying down because their eustachian tubes are not draining. If you prop the head up while sleeping or just sit up for a few minutes, you can sometimes ease the pain.

Avoid the smoke screen

There is a well-documented link between parental smoking and childhood ear infection. If you as a parent smoke, stop, not just for your own sake, but for your child's. Also, do whatever you can to prevent your child from getting second hand smoke from others.

Vacuum therapy

Tests have shown that rugs and carpets are approximately twenty times (!) dirtier than the average city sidewalk. An infant's or child's allergy leading to an earache can be set off by the dirt and dust in a rug, especially if the children spend much time crawling or playing on the floor. Vacuum frequently.

Pacify infants during air travel

Infants tend to experience great distress during air travel due to the inadequate opening of the eustachian tube during the rapid change in air pressure. To prevent this problem, infants should be nursed, or given a pacifier or bottle during takeoff and landing.

FATIGUE
▼

Fatigue can make everything more difficult. Remote control for television is a godsend for the seriously fatigued but, unfortunately, there is no remote control for most of life's other activities.

Fatigue is a frustrating condition; not only does it affect your physical energy but it affects your mental energy too. Symptoms that commonly accompany fatigue are the inability to think clearly, sleep disturbances, constipation, apathy, depression, swollen glands, and difficulty readinginginging.

Chronic fatigue syndrome has become the latest garbage-can diagnosis for various fatigue-related health problems. Some physicians think that it is caused by the Epstein-Barr virus, others think it's from the HBLV virus, and still others think that it's a mixture (or cocktail) of several viruses.

Some fatigue syndromes have nothing to do with viral infection but could be the result of anemia, a thyroid problem, or some other condition. And some fatigue syndromes result from psychological problems, although, in these cases, it is often difficult to determine if the psychological problem caused the fatigue or if the fatigue led to the psychological problem.

Fatigue can be caused by overexertion, but it can also result

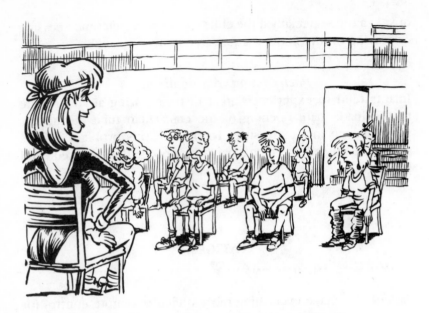

"Okay, everyone, lift that right eyelid, and close it . . .
now the left eyelid . . ."
Aerobics for the Seriously Fatigued

from underexertion. A couch potato is as likely to become fatigued as an overstressed athlete.

The fact that you've read this far means you're not a total basketcase. Here are some strategies to get you up, on your feet again, and raring to go.

Energy creates energy

Exercise may sound impossible when you're fatigued, but it does stimulate circulation and metabolism. Regular exercise usually enhances energy; just be careful not to exhaust yourself.

Take a cold shower

This strategy will wake you up. If you're not brave enough to do this, take a cold foot bath, or simply splash your face with cold water.

Avoid cheap tricks

Drinking coffee and eating sweets may give you short-term energy, but they can lead to greater fatigue because these substances sap the adrenal glands and disrupt blood-sugar levels. Stay away from these energy-robbers.

Go light on lunch

Large lunch meals, especially those with high-fat foods, commonly cause afternoon fatigue. Avoid them unless it is okay for you to sleep at your desk.

Watch your protein

Fatigue can result from having too much protein or too little. Make certain you're getting enough, but not too much. One meal per day, maybe two at the most, should have a food that is rich with protein. Meat and dairy products are sources of protein, but there are healthier alternatives. You can get complete protein meals with less fat by eating plenty of whole grains, vegetables, legumes, and seeds.

Start the day right

It is best to have a good breakfast. Whole grain cereals (oatmeal for example) have plenty of natural carbohydrates that provide sustained energy.

Are your drugs putting you to sleep?

Fatigue and tiredness are common side effects of various prescription and over-the-counter drugs. Sleeping pills may help you fall asleep, but they commonly lead to increased fatigue the next day. Other energy-drainers are high blood pressure drugs and cold and cough medicines.

Warm your liver

A heating pad placed over your lower right ribcage for twenty minutes twice a day can increase liver activity and help your body digest sugars better, creating more energy.

Make the most of your good times
Some people with fatigue find that they have more energy at specific times of the day or night. Make use of these times to do your more intensive tasks and to practice healing efforts.

Supplement your energy
Take vitamin C three times a day, beta-carotene, B-complex, and vitamin E twice a day, and chelated magnesium, chelated zinc, and calcium once per day. If you take these supplements with your meals they will be easier to assimilate.

Herbal interferon
Echinacea is an herb that has been proven to be effective in reducing viral activity. It also stimulates the immune system, and some people with fatigue who take it have noticed improved energy and stamina. Take fifteen drops of *echinacea* tincture three times a day.

Take advantage of your slowed-down condition
Savor every short-term activity. Appreciate the little things in life. Read a paragraph and truly digest it. Meditate for twenty minutes, and try to do it twice a day. Try yoga; the exercises won't exhaust you, and they can help to oxygenate your cells in a gentle way.

Try aggressive rest therapy
The body is better able to heal itself during sleep. Get an adequate amount of sleep, and take naps as needed during the day without feeling guilty about it. As you close your eyes, affirm your sleeping and napping times as healing experiences.

Try aggressive emotional rest too
Don't waste your energy on negative emotions. All they do is drain you and add to your fatigue. When you're fatigued you tend to complain about it; that's expected, but watch yourself to make certain you don't dwell on complaining. Also, try not to get sucked into other people's emotional dramas, unless you can get

in and out without exhausting yourself. You have enough of your own dramas to worry about.

Forgive yourself; forgive others

When you're fatigued, you may not be able to keep up your regular can-do attitude. Allow yourself to lick your wounds and heal yourself. Forgive others who may not understand why you don't have the energy to do things the way you've done them in the past.

Take your job and love it

If you truly love your work it can be the best energizer for you. Anything that gives your life purpose and meaning is highly therapeutic. If you're unable to change jobs to one that you feel passionate about, do whatever you can to turn your present job into one that you love.

HEADACHES (MIGRAINE)
.... ▼ ....

It is accurate to tell a person with a migraine that the pain is all in their head. Considering that a migraine sufferer's head usually feels like it is the size of a city block, that's a lot of pain.

During a migraine headache, blood vessels first become overly constricted, then abnormally widened. You usually experience this pain on one side of your head, which can make you feel lopsided.

Migraines are often triggered by psychological stress, but unlike tension headaches, migraines tend to begin after a stressed person is finally able to relax; then that relaxing weekend or vacation becomes relaxation hell.

Other triggers of migraines are sleeping too long, bright lights, too much time between eating, and fluctuations in hormone levels (some women get migraines during menstruation or ovulation). Certain foods, drinks, and drugs can also set off a migraine.

When a migraine is triggered, your head seems to explode. It feels like there's an alien being in there trying to get out through your eyes. It feels like there's someone knocking at a door inside your head, and no one is home to answer, so the knocking just goes on. These are but some of the exciting experiences inside the torture chamber of a migraine sufferer's head.

Some migraine sufferers experience symptoms that warn them of an impending headache. Most commonly, these warning symptoms are disturbances of vision, slurred speech, dizziness, floating visual images, or weakness or numbness of one side of the body. If you are having a headache or any of these warning symptoms (and it's not from drinking alcohol), consider these strategies.

Loosen up
Family therapist Virginia Satir once said, "If you have a stiff body, it's no wonder you're numb upstairs." Loosen your body. Try to move every joint in your body, one joint at a time, through its full range of motion. If you have access to a pool, do it in water.

Around your head in a couple of minutes
While sitting up, relax your head and allow it to be as limp as possible, letting your chin touch, or almost touch, your upper chest. Rotate your head clockwise *very slowly* several times and then counter-clockwise the same number of times.

Get moving
Exercise can be effective in preventing a migraine. When you feel a headache coming on, exercise it out of you. If it hurts to move too much, try gentle motion exercise such as yoga, tai chi, or slow swimming.

Headache-few with feverfew
New research published in the *Lancet* has shown that the herb feverfew is very helpful for vascular headaches. Scientists have

proven that feverfew stops the blood platelets from releasing an excessive amount of serotonin, which seems to be one of the causes of migraines. Make an herbal tea of it, or simply take a feverfew capsule.

Don't feed your head(ache)

Certain foods can trigger a vascular headache. No food will cause *everybody's* headache, but many migraine sufferers recognize that there are foods that do aggravate their problem. The most common offenders are nuts, chocolate, coffee, sauerkraut, wheat, cheese and other dairy products, hot dogs, luncheon meats that contain nitrites, citrus, MSG, and alcohol (especially red wine).

As above, so below

The congestion you feel in your head may be connected, in part, to the congestion you feel in your gut. Read Constipation section.

As below, so above

Stand on your head or shoulders, or hang upside down. Remember to breathe regularly. This exercise stimulates circulation and helps to break up head congestion. Do this for a minute, and then, with practice, try to extend it. To avoid possible head or neck injury, you should learn the proper position from a yoga book or yoga practitioner. Don't do it if you have back problems or if it makes your head hurt too much.

Hot bathing and cold-water torture

Fill a bathtub with hot water and add several teaspoons of Epsom salts. Soak in the tub for ten to twenty minutes; melt and relax in this comfort. Dry off, drain the water, get back in the tub, and take a cold shower for about three minutes. Dry off, dress in warm bedclothes, and relax in bed. This strategy is not for everyone; some people are hypersensitive during headaches to heat or cold. If you can stand to do this hot and cold bathing, you'll receive the benefits of improved circulation, and reduced head congestion and head pain.

Learn to circulate

With the aid of biofeedback, you can learn to directly affect blood circulation in your body, including the head congestion of a migraine headache. Courses in biofeedback are often available at community colleges, hospitals, and health centers.

Magnesium magic

Magnesium relaxes the constriction of blood vessels and helps to lower blood pressure. Some studies have shown that 200 mg. of magnesium helps relieve migraines. Try taking this dose three times a day with meals.

Have sex!

Although some people use headaches as an excuse for *not* having sex, a researcher at Southern Illinois University has found that sex may actually provide some relief for migraine sufferers. The researcher found that the more intense the orgasm, the more intense the relief.

Read and try some of the strategies for tension headaches too.

One useless idea

Two-thirds of all people who suffer from migraines come from a family of fellow sufferers. Because changing one's parents is not a practical strategy, it is best to consider the previous strategies.

HEADACHES (TENSION)

▼

Approximately 90 percent of all headaches are tension headaches. Perhaps they should be called "tension neck- and backaches" because it's the tightening of the neck and back muscles that usually creates the head pain. The old Persian proverb that says,

"The bigger a man's head, the worse his headache," may be correct after all—the extra weight on the neck and the extra ego that comes with a swollen head may be enough to make anyone feel top heavy.

Tension headaches seem to be an equal opportunity affliction. They can be caused by almost any type of stress: too much or too little exertion, too much or too little excitement, too hot or too cold temperature, too much or too little sleep, too erect or too limp posture, too much or too little food, and so on.

A tension headache can lead to irresponsible behavior. Even this, though, may have a practical value. It allows you to tell your spouse, "I can't do the dishes, honey." You can tell your employer, "I can't finish that project." You can tell your children, "Shut up and stop having fun." This selfish behavior, of course, should lead you to rest and take care of your headache. Sometimes, it seems that a headache is nature's way of telling you to relax.

If, however, your teeth are clenched so tightly that people think you're doing your Clint Eastwood impersonation, and if your eyeballs hurt when you move them, even across this page, then you are paying the price of not resting and enjoying yourself enough. You now have some catching-up to do.

(If your eyes are not cooperating with you, get someone to read the following strategies to you.)

Don't relax . . . at least not yet
An effective technique for reducing tension headaches is to tighten the muscles in the head, neck, and jaw for five to ten seconds . . . and then release them. You may find that you will be able to achieve a deep level of relaxation and relief from this simple exercise.

Get in touch with the temples
Remember the old aspirin commercials showing a furrow-browed man with an awful headache? As you may recall, he is seen massaging his temples. There are important acupressure points at the

temples which can be used to relieve tension. Place four fingers (not the thumb) along both temples and do a circular massaging motion. Massage for a minute ... and call me in the morning.

Head to acupressure
The head and neck are full of invaluable acupressure points that can release tension when they are pressed firmly. Search your head and neck for hot points, that is, points that seem to be sensitive to pressure. Press them for at least five seconds, then relax for five seconds. Repeat several times.

Your head is in your hands
There is an acupuncture point just barely under the bottom of the nail of your middle finger. If the pain is primarily on one side, then press the point on the hand of that side. If it's on both sides, then alternate pressing this point on each hand.

Pretend to yawn
Chew a bit. Relax that jaw! If your jaw is tense, muscles in your head and neck can impede blood-flow to the head and aggravate tension headaches.

Run away
Exercise can help loosen you up and release head, neck, and back tension. Exercising outside, as long as it is not too smoggy, carries the extra health benefit of breathing fresh air.

Take a break from your coffee break
Drinking coffee is known to cause headaches in many people. It is also common to experience headaches while going through caffeine withdrawal. Don't drink coffee; break away from it.

Head for the herbs
Various herbal teas can help you to relax. Place a tablespoon each of chamomile and scullcap into a cup of boiling water and let steep for five minutes. Another good combination of herbs is one

teaspoon each of hops and peppermint, and two teaspoons each of chamomile, rosemary, and wood betony.

A bright idea
Cool-white fluorescent lights—which are commonly used in many businesses—give some people headaches. Ask your employer to help enhance worker health and productivity by replacing these bulbs with full-spectrum lighting.

Color yourself pain-free
Close your eyes and imagine a cool color pervading your head and neck. Choose whatever color is soothing to you. This cooling color should be moving and sweeping around; don't let it stagnate. Research has shown that color does affect brain chemistry and behavior. Color therapy is not simply something for those who are interested in fashion; it also has potentially profound healing effects.

No noise is good noise
Excessive noise can irritate anyone. Avoid loud music or being in situations where there is a lot of noise.

See if your head is on straight
"_____ (your name), sit up straight!" Improper posture can put stress on neck and back muscles. If your office chair, your car's seat, or any chair in your house doesn't give you good support, do something about it.

Learn to listen to your body
One of the most common and effective uses of biofeedback is teaching people how to treat headaches by learning how to consciously relax head, neck, and jaw muscles. After you master some basics of the ability to affect your own body, you can learn to do so without being hooked up to a machine.

Watch Candid Camera *reruns*

Laughter releases tension. You may laugh your headache off.

Play a different game

Tension headaches can result from an over-competitive personality. Create win–win situations. Appreciate the art of losing. Honor quality of performance, not the prize.

HEART DISEASE

▼

Heart disease is the number one killer of men and women in western civilization, primarily because we are accomplices to

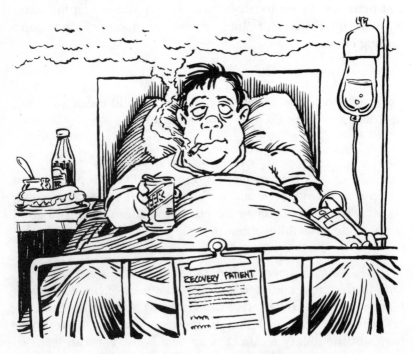

Bypass surgery tends to bypass the problem.

this crime. Our high-fat diet, sedentary lifestyle, stressful environment, and various vices—tobacco, alcohol, and recreational drugs—harden the heart and its arteries, and increase the risk of heart disease and early death.

In addition to these negative influences that weigh heavily on the heart, we also tend to suffer from a deficiency in the positive experiences that lighten the heart's load. Love, joy, pleasure, humor, and other enriching feelings not only help us feel joyfully connected with others but also may help to keep open the arteries and veins so that our circulatory system is able to connect with all parts of our body in a healthy way.

There are many influences that increase or decrease your risk of heart disease, though, like so many issues in medicine and science, there is probably more controversy than agreement on what exactly you should do to help yourself live a longer, healthier life. Even when the "experts" agree on some issue, it is always uncertain how long the agreement will last. There was, for instance, some consensus that salt was a significant factor in hypertension. Recent research, however, has shown that salt does not lead to hypertension in most people, only those who are, for unknown reasons, sensitive to it.

Despite the controversies and ambiguities of medical science, it is instructive to remember the words of Norman Cousins, who said, "No one knows enough to be a pessimist about their own health." On this optimistic note, I encourage you to consider the following strategies, which hopefully will not only help you lead a longer, healthier life but a more joyful one as well.

Flex those heart muscles

Exercise! Medical associations usually encourage heart patients to consult their physician before beginning an exercise program. Considering the therapeutic value of exercise upon the heart and a person's overall health, it seems more wise to see a physician if you choose *not* to exercise. A sedentary lifestyle should only be available by prescription to people with a serious disorder. The best form of exercise for a healthy heart is one which exercises the long muscles, such as jogging, swimming, rowing, walking, and running sports. Isometrics and weightlifting, on the other hand, can raise your blood pressure and should be avoided.

Lighten up

Jog with a fifty-pound backpack. After a minute or so you will rapidly discover what extra stress this extra baggage has put on you and your heart. If you're not at or near your optimal weight level, you are continually putting extra stress on your heart. One option: if you simply maintain your present calorie intake for one year and increase your activity level by walking one mile a day, you will lose ten pounds.

Pretend you're Italian

Put garlic on everything. Garlic has been shown to prevent the formation of clots, to lower blood pressure, to reduce plaque formation, and even to reverse established atherosclerosis. Garlic also boosts the high-density lipoproteins (the good guys!). Brave people or hermits should try eating fresh cloves; others can purchase the capsulated garlic.

Sow your oats (and other sources of fiber)

The water-soluble fiber from various grains, especially oats, is able to get into your arteries, break down cholesterol, and do some roto-rooter style cleaning. Psyllium, the primary ingredient in Metamucil, has been found to significantly lower serum cholesterol. Most whole grains and legumes are good sources of fiber, especially wheat, brown rice, lentils, and dried peas. Most fresh fruits and vegetables, especially apples, figs, broccoli, and brussels sprouts are also good sources.

Hearty supplements

The following supplements can be helpful to the heart: 100 to 400 IU of vitamin E three times a day, 1,000 to 3,000 mg. of vitamin C, 200 mcg. a day of chromium picolinate,100 mcg. a day of selenium, and 500 to 1,000 mg. of calcium (calcium is especially important for post-menopausal women). Magnesium and potassium supplements are particularly important if you're taking diuretics.

Niacin to the rescue
Niacin has been shown to lower the amount of bad cholesterol in the body and increase the amount of good cholesterol. A decrease of ten to twenty-five percent in cholesterol is common in people who either take niacin alone or with other supplements. It is recommended to increase the amount of niacin slowly. Start with 100 mg. of niacin three times a day for the first three days, increase to 200 mg. three times a day for the next three days, and then increase by 100 mg. per dose every three days until you are taking 1,000 mg. per dose three times a day. Niacin should not, however, be taken if you have liver disease.

Cut the fat out
If you have heart disease, just cutting a little fat out of your diet is not really going to help. To make real headway and heartway, you've got to seriously cut down on *all* fats, especially animal fats. It is particularly important to avoid eating late at night when whatever fat you eat goes into the bloodstream at a time when your circulation has slowed down, leading to increased chances of arterial blockage.

It's tea time!
Black tea contains tannic acid, an astringent compound that has been found to lower cholesterol. Do not, however, brew your black tea too long; taking too large a dose of it can lead to indigestion.

To aspirin or not to aspirin
Although recent research has shown the benefits of aspirin to the heart, other research has shown that aspirin can have detrimental effects upon the immune system. Aspirin not only blocks the anti-clotting effects of hormone-like chemicals called prostaglandins,

but it also inhibits the infection-fighting action of the prostaglandins. There are safer means of preventing heart disease. If you do decide to use aspirin to prevent blood clotting and a heart attack, only take half an aspirin a day.

Relax and relax again

Do whatever activities relax you, and consider using tried-and-true strategies such as meditation, yoga, and biofeedback that can help you obtain deeper states of relaxation. Just as many people go to aerobics classes to help them maintain a fitness program, it is likewise helpful to go regularly to yoga, meditation, or relaxation classes. The expert teaching and group support will help keep you on the program better than if you do it alone.

Relaxation is only a breath away

Proper breathing is not only relaxing, it can help oxygenate the blood and improve heart function. Most people breathe primarily with their chest which encourages rapid and shallow breathing. A deeper and more relaxing breath is obtained through abdominal breathing. To practice abdominal breathing, sit comfortably with your back straight. Place one hand on your chest and the other on your abdomen. Breathing in through your nose, notice the hand on your abdomen rise, while the hand on your chest hardly moves. Exhale as much as possible, even contracting your abdominal muscles so that they slightly massage the internal organs. Breathe in again through your nose. Repeat this process for a couple of minutes, several times a day. Although this type of breathing will feel uncomfortable at first, doing it more frequently will teach you to breathe more deeply, helping you to relax more fully and to improve your health.

Drink an herbal cocktail

Make a tea of hawthorn berries (one teaspoon of berries per cup of water); then add a pinch of cayenne and a clove of garlic. Hawthorn berries are a cardiac tonic which has antispasmoidic and sedative action as well. They can help lower blood pressure, regulate heart beat, and prevent clotting. If the berries themselves are unavailable, go to a health food store to obtain either the liquid form (take twenty to forty drops twice a day) or the powdered, encapsulated form (two capsules twice a day). The cayenne helps distribute the healing effects of the hawthorn berries and garlic throughout your circulatory system.

Get hot, get cool
Stimulate circulation by alternating hot showers and cool showers. Do three minutes of each twice. As your heart and your courage strengthen, try using even colder and hotter water. If you're in a drought area, consider other strategies.

Try pleasure therapy
Do whatever you truly love, not just because it feels good, but because it's also therapeutic.

The healing power of work
Work satisfaction is invaluable to a healthy heart. If your work is fulfilling you, this satisfaction warms the heart and lowers the blood pressure. Recent research has also shown that people whose job is not secure are more apt to have higher levels of serum cholesterol and higher rates of heart attack.

Friendship therapy
Research has shown that people with social support networks tend to suffer less from heart disease. Call and visit a friend just for the heart of it.

Acknowledge fear; release it
The emotion of fear is a primordial survival defense; it prepares you for fight or flight. However, fear also raises your blood pressure, and if you experience it for a prolonged period of time, it can lead to hypertension. Because we sometimes feel fear when neither a fight or flight response is appropriate, we are often bottling up powerful emotions and disturbing our health. If you

try to ignore your fears they fester, while acknowledging them is the first step that helps bring light to the darkness. As Gandolf, one of the heroes in *The Hobbit* said, "We must go in the direction of our greatest fear, for therein lies our only hope." Because fear often raises its head when we ignore its roots, when we seek to understand it we help release it.

HEMORRHOIDS
▼

William Blake once wrote, "Expect poison from standing waters." Blake's words were not intended to provide insight linking constipation and hemorrhoids, and yet, with apologies to the poet, it can be said that the standing waters of constipation create the breeding grounds for various health problems, including hemorrhoids.

Hemorrhoids occur when the veins at the anus are overly stretched as the result of excessive pressure, usually from straining during the passage of stools. These bulging veins can occur at the anus wall or the lower bowel. When this bulging occurs in the lower bowel, the hemorrhoid is not visible to the eye and is thus called a *blind hemorrhoid*. Obesity, inactivity, frequent use of laxatives, and anal intercourse can also contribute to hemorrhoids.

Hemorrhoids are one of the most common afflictions in western civilization. More than half of all Americans will suffer from this undignified malady at least once in their life. Its most common symptom is rectal bleeding, which is usually discovered by noticing blood on the toilet paper or blood-streaked stools. Hemorrhoids, not suprisingly, are often a pain in the butt, including soreness, burning, and itching, though many people do not experience any pain at all.

Surgery is sometimes performed on people with severe cases, but such drastic treatment doesn't change the factors which led to hemorrhoids in the first place. It has been said that "a hatchet is a good thing, but not for eating soup." Likewise, surgery is a good thing, but ...

People with hemorrhoids who do not rise up to do something to heal themselves may be forced to sit on their problem. Here are some strategies to try before you raise the hatchet.

Read the Constipation chapter!
Eat your fiber first.

Drink up
Drink lots of fluids, especially water. If you don't, that extra fiber that you should be taking may actually aggravate your constipation.

Witch hazel isn't a witch
Witch hazel is an herb (*Hamamelis*) which is a tried-and-true folk remedy for hemorrhoids. Distilled witch hazel is available at most drug stores and is applied externally. Witch hazel can also be taken as a suppository. It is also available as a homeopathic ointment in many health-food stores and some pharmacies.

Don't just sit there
It may be karmic justice that it is sometimes painful to sit when you have hemorrhoids. Since this condition can be aggravated by physical inactivity, the pain from sitting is a painfully clear message that you should get off your duff and exercise.

Don't read on the throne
Because people who are constipated sometimes take a long time to defecate, they often bring a book or a magazine with them. Although reading may help pass the time, it doesn't necessarily help anything else pass and may, in fact, increase the time it takes. Since sitting for prolonged periods can aggravate hemorrhoids, leave *War and Peace* for your reading chair, not the toilet.

Don't stop breathing
When the going gets tough, people tend to stop breathing in their efforts to push out a stool. This straining can aggravate hemorrhoids. It is better to breathe deeply and evenly during bowel movements.

Schizophrenic bathing
Alternate taking a hot bath and a cold bath of twenty minutes each. Only your lower abdomen, hips, and buttocks should be immersed. The alternating of hot and cold water stimulates circulation.

Internal herbal relief
Stoneroot (*Collinsonia canadensis*) and pilewort (*lesser celandine*) are herbs which have been used for hemorrhoids for thousands of years. If it was good for you in a past life, it may be good for you today. Take two capsules of either of these herbs with a glass of water twice a day or place one ounce of the herb in one pint of boiling water. Let it steep and drink one-half cup twice a day.

External herbal relief
Yarrow (*Millefolium*) and golden seal (*Hydrastis*) are both astringent herbs, which means that they can constrict the bulging tissue of hemorrhoids. Steep yarrow, and then add a teaspoon of golden seal powder. Take a cotton swab and apply it directly to the afflicted area.

Supplementary relief
Take 1,000 to 2,000 mg. of vitamin C, 400 IU of vitamin E, 25,000 IU of vitamin A and potassium, 600 mg. of calcium and 300 mg. of magnesium. Vitamins C and E strengthen capillaries, vitamin A improves the integrity of cell walls, and potassium, calcium, and magnesium are vital for muscle health. If much blood is lost from the hemorrhoid, take 10 to 15 mg. of iron, 400 mcg. of folic acid and 1 to 4 mcg. of B_{12}.

Take preparation H-omeopathic

You might, however, consider taking a small dose of a substance which would cause hemorrhoids if taken in a larger (non-homeopathic) dose. Homeopathic *Hamamelis* (witch hazel) *12* or *30* is good for bleeding hemorrhoids that cause a bruised soreness, possibly with pulsations felt in the rectum. *Aesculus* (horse chestnut) *12* or *30* is good for hemorrhoidal pain that is made worse by standing or walking, usually without bleeding and sometimes with a backache. This medicine is commonly given to women who have hemorrhoids during menopause. *Pulsatilla* (windflower) *12* or *30* is good for blind hemorrhoids with itching and sticking pains, especially in pregnant women. *Nux vomica* (poison nut) *12* or *30* is good for blind hemorrhoids in people who have frequent ineffectual urgings for a bowel movement, often because of abuse of laxatives or various drugs.

A yogic tune-up

Tone your abdomen by lying on your back with your feet flat on the floor. Place your feet close to your buttocks, and lift your hips off the floor. Take a complete breath in and out while remaining in the raised position. Raise and lower yourself six times in this way.

Some things not to do

Avoid prolonged use of laxatives or mineral oil (even herbal laxatives). Avoid using ointments and suppositories for more than fourteen days unless your condition is medically monitored. Avoid scratching the irritated area and avoid heavy lifting.

HERPES

▼

Herpes was once considered the modern scarlet letter, until the AIDS epidemic spread and stole its thunder. Although this sexually-transmitted disease is no longer a media star, herpes is as common, perhaps even more so, than it was several years ago, and it is just as problematic for the infected person.

Herpes, like AIDS and the common cold, is caused by a virus, and it is presently believed that once you are infected, the virus will always inhabit your body. Although you may be horrified by this prospect, it generally is not as traumatic as it sounds. Many people who get infected experience only a single eruption and rarely or never get another. Even for those people who get more frequent eruptions, modern medical drugs and some emerging natural therapies can be very effective in reducing the frequency and intensity of outbreaks.

Herpetic eruptions most commonly occur on the lips, around the mouth, or on the genitals, though they are each caused by different viruses. Herpes of the mouth is caused by herpesvirus Type 1, and herpes of the genitals by herpesvirus Type 2. (For the first time in medical history, names of a virus are comprehendable by the average patient.) Strangely enough, the popular name of mouth herpes is confusingly called both a "cold sore" and a "fever blister." Perhaps people can't figure out if this eruption is too cold or too hot.

Although the herpes condition can be relatively benign, it can cause complications when a pregnant woman with an herpetic outbreak gives birth because the infant can get a potentially fatal infection. Herpes has also been linked to later onset of cervical cancer. Furthermore, if herpes is spread to the eye, it can lead to blindness. (People who get such infections may be looking for love in all the wrong places.)

Perhaps the most frequent complication of herpes is the guilt and general anxiety that too often accompany this infection. Those infected with herpes often observe that they are more prone to outbreaks during psychological stress, thus the more they reduce their extra baggage of anxieties, the less they have to experience the discomfort of herpes.

New research has developed a herpes vaccine, but only for mice. Although this vaccine may mean little for current sufferers, such advances may be invaluable in the future. For now, here are a few strategies to help alleviate some of the pain and discomfort of herpes.

Freeze 'em out
If you apply ice to herpes sores as soon as they erupt, you can sometimes prevent them from getting worse.

Witch hazel to the rescue
Apply distilled witch hazel to sores to help dry them out. Another herb that can dry out herpes blisters is tincture of myrrh.

A blow-dryer job
Another way to dry out moist blisters is to use a blow-dryer. Be careful though not to irritate the sores by blow-drying too long or too closely.

Take tea and see
Pour a little hot water over a black tea bag—just enough to moisten it—then set the tea bag aside for a couple minutes. After it cools down, place the tea bag on the sore. Black tea has tannic acid which not only can reduce the pain, but is an astringent that can help constrict the skin.

Red wine will make it fine
Researchers have found that freeze-dried red wine has concentrated tannins in it which can relieve the pain of herpes sores. Apply it topically with a cotton swab. Freeze-dried red wine is available in some wine specialty shops.

Salt your wounds
Add one-half cup of salt to your bath water and sit in it. This may sting a bit at first but you will soon feel relief.

Check your aminos
Some research has shown that increasing certain amino acids and decreasing others leads to reduced and less intense herpetic erup-

tions. You should determine for yourself if this program helps. The amino acid lysine may help to inhibit herpes replication, while another amino acid, arginine, encourages herpes replication. Increase lysine by taking a supplement separate from a meal (1,000 mg. a day when sores aren't active and 2,000 mg. when they are active) and/or eating more of the following foods: fish (especially shark), chicken, milk, yogurt, fresh vegetables, eggs, Brewers yeast, soybeans, and legumes. Because sugar, fats, and protein can inhibit absorption of lysine, it is wise to reduce their consumption. Foods rich in arginine which should be avoided are nuts, chocolate, seeds, cottonseed oil, coconut, macaroni, oats, wheatgerm, whole wheat bread, and coffee.

External vitamins
Open a capsule of vitamin E and apply the liquid directly to the sores every four hours.

Don't touch yourself
Avoid touching your sores, but if you do, wash your hands carefully afterwards so that you don't spread the virus to other parts of your body, especially your eyes.

Let your skin breathe
Wear natural-fiber clothing that allows skin to breathe, and avoid pants and underwear that are too tight. Also, avoid applying petroleum jelly and antibiotic ointments which inhibit the ability of your skin to breathe and can slow the healing of herpes blisters.

Soothing herbs
Tinctures of *Calendula* (marigold) and *Hypericum* (St. John's wort) are both soothing herbs which can reduce some of the inflammation of a herpes sore.

The healing powers of poison ivy
Believe it or not, poison ivy—in a homeopathic dose—is often effective in treating people with herpes. Because poison ivy can

cause blisters that resemble herpes, utilizing the principles of homeopathy, very small doses of poison ivy can help heal them. Use *Rhus tox* (poison ivy) *6* or *30* three times a day for two or three days. Another helpful homeopathic medicine to try is *Natrum mur* (salt) *6* or *30*.

Avoid heavy sex
Even when you do not have an eruption, vigorous or longlasting sex can irritate the genitals and cause eruptions. This is particularly a problem if partners are not adequately lubricated.

Condomize
Using condoms is important in preventing infection in others. Because it is possible to spread herpes even when you don't have an obvious sore, it's best to use them every time you have sex. (There are, of course, a few other good reasons.)

Get support
Join a herpes support group if you feel you need help in working out whatever feelings of guilt, fear, or anxiety you experience because of your condition.

You are not herpes
You may have herpes, but that doesn't mean you *are* herpes. Avoid identifying yourself, even subconsciously, as a herpes person. This attitude may not cure your herpes, but it will reduce the anxieties that tend to accompany the outbreaks.

INDIGESTION
▼

Some people say you are what you eat, but, since we don't digest all the food we eat, the saying should be, "you are what you assimilate." However, even this perspective is narrowly focussed

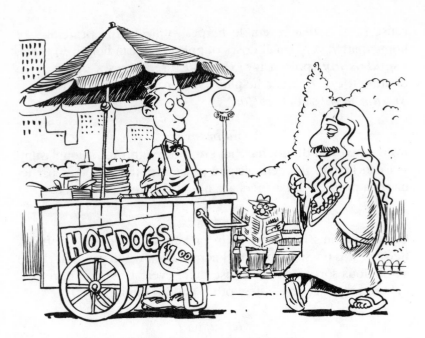

"Make me one with everything."
Zen master about to become one with indigestion.

on food. If you are what your body takes in, are you then also what you breathe, what your skin absorbs, and what your mind thinks? If we are all this and more, mixed together, it is certainly understandable why so many people have indigestion.

Indigestion is a very broad term that refers to virtually any problem with digesting food. Most commonly, it refers to heartburn, gas, and distention of the abdomen (see sections on Constipation, Diarrhea, Irritable bowel syndrome, Nausea and Vomiting, and Ulcers for information on each of these related conditions).

Heartburn is a misnomer, since it is not really the heart that is burning. Perhaps it's called this because it is often the food we truly love that tends to upset us, thus breaking our heart—and our stomach. Heartburn is actually a condition in which the esophagus or stomach is irritated by too much acid from the foods we have eaten or from the digestive acids that are secreted to digest them. The body may slightly regurgitate the food and the acids, thereby creating some burning in the middle of the chest. Because the pain is at or near the heart, heartburn is scary, leading many to take over-the-counter medications that provide temporary relief. These drugs, however, offer only short-term relief and often aggravate the condition.

Stomach gas is experienced by virtually everyone, though some people are larger producers of it than others. This gas can come from excessive swallowing of air or from the action of bacteria due to the incomplete digestion of carbohydrates. Depending on where the gas is temporarily trapped, the body will release it through one orifice or another. And remember that over two thousand years ago, Hippocrates said that "passing gas is necessary to well-being."

In the 1960s, a classic commercial showed a man talking to his stomach. His stomach expressed concern about the way the man was treating it and asked the man to be more sensitive to its problems. Whether you talk to your stomach or not, your stomach talks to you. It talks to you by the way it expresses its symptoms. Sometimes its message is clear and direct—"Stop eating that food," "Don't eat any more," "Eat more slowly," while at other times it is difficult to interpret what it is saying. You may ask yourself: Which food should I stop eating? Why do I have gas now? That antacid worked before, why isn't it working now?

We were all taught to speak at least one language, and sometimes several, but few of us have learned to understand the language of the body. And even if we know what the body is saying, we don't always pay attention.

Whether we understand what our bodies are saying or not, it is worthwhile to listen. It is also worthwhile to ask the body what it means. Since the body doesn't speak English, "asking it" may mean testing it by doing or eating something different, then paying attention to the reaction. Here are some strategies to experiment with in your efforts to respond to your poor, abused digestive system.

Eat small

Don't be stuck in the habit of eating three large meals a day. Eating smaller, more frequent meals is a great way to reduce indigestion.

Slow down and chew

One more instance in which your parents were right! A significant percentage of digestion, especially of carbohydrates, takes place in your mouth from juices in the saliva. If you gulp down your food, you're not giving your body enough opportunity to digest it. You should try to chew your foods until they're almost liquid in your mouth. You should even chew your drinks, especially juices and sodas. By holding a drink in your mouth and chewing several times you mix in salivary digestive enzymes which enable you to digest the juice or soda more effectively. Just remember: drink your food and chew your drinks.

Slow the fiber

Although fiber is important for digestion and elimination, too much fiber or a too rapid increase of fiber in the diet can cause serious gas problems. The foods with the most fiber are bran, prunes, figs, whole grains, legumes, broccoli, cauliflower, onions, cabbage, and raisins.

Avoid heartburn hotel

Coffee, acidic fruits (tomatoes and grapefruits), chocolate, alcohol, nitrates, and fatty foods can irritate the lining of the esophagus and lead to heartburn. Even smoking can cause heartburn because it increases pressure at the lower end of the esophagus.

Get the right combination

Some people notice that they develop indigestion if they eat certain foods in combination. This may be true for you. Some of the most common problem combinations are a meat dish eaten with a starchy food or a grain dish eaten with dairy products. Some people also experience digestive problems when they eat fruit with any other food. The good news here is that you may discover that a food that had previously caused you digestive problems may be fine as long as it is not combined with other foods.

Avoid the bubbly

Carbonated drinks and beer can create or add to a gas problem. Since you can't bottle the gas you create, it's better to avoid these drinks.

Artificial sweetener creates not-so-artificial problems

Artificial sweeteners are nondigestable carbohydrates that turn your body into a gas machine. Avoid them.

Milk can add fuel to the flames

Milk and dairy products can aggravate heartburn because the body must produce increased acid to digest them.

Suck up to a straw

Drinking through a straw cuts down on the air that you may be inhaling as you drink.

Bring out the charcoal

Activated charcoal tablets are invaluable for excessive flatulence since charcoal absorbs gas.

Don't take it lying down

People with chronic heartburn should not eat while reclining or lying down. In fact, you should avoid lying down until two or three hours after eating.

An oat and bran cocktail

Soak one tablespoon each of oatmeal and bran in a pint of water for thirty minutes. Strain and drink the water. This liquid is both nourishing and soothing to the digestive tract.

An old-time remedy
A tablespoon of apple cider vinegar before meals is an old-time remedy for acid indigestion. A tablespoon each of apple cider vinegar and honey is also great for relieving gas.

In mint condition
Peppermint and spearmint tea are soothing for many types of indigestion. Other herbal teas that are digestion-helpers are chamomile, rosemary, and blackberry.

More herbal help
Fennel seeds are commonly available at the counters of Indian restaurants because they are known to help you digest food better. One special recipe to augment the action of fennel is to grind it and add it to a mixture of grated ginger and honey. Eat it with a spoon. It tastes great and it's good for you. Also, slippery elm bark—one-quarter of an ounce to a pint of water—is a wonderfully soothing and nourishing drink for the digestive system. (I must warn you that this mixture is rather slimy and tastes a bit weird!)

A spicy digestive aid
Garlic is invaluable both for painful digestion and for flatulence.

The drugs made you do it
Certain prescription drugs cause indigestion. Check with your doctor about the drugs that you are taking; you may want to avoid these drugs or switch to others.

Relieve pressure by placing pressure
While holding the two sides of your knee cap with your index finger and thumb, place your middle finger outside of the shin bone and press it for five to ten seconds. This acupressure point is Stomach 36 and applying pressure to it can relax the stomach and reduce indigestion.

142

Sit-ups for health

Sit-ups improve abdominal muscle tone and can reduce excessive distention. Do them regularly.

Relax during those private moments

Straining during defecation can increase abdominal pressure, causing heartburn and indigestion. Take it slow and easy.

Bottle up the belching

Forced belching tends to add even more air to the stomach than it releases. Not only is forced belching ill-mannered, it isn't good for you.

Release the butterflies in your stomach

Accept the anxiety, the nervousness, and the fear that you are holding in, then release it. If you need to scream, scream. If you need to jump around, jump around. If you need to talk incessantly, do so ... but only if you can find a receptive listener.

INFLUENZA

Also called *the grippe*, influenza can indeed get a strong hold on you. It can last for seven to ten days and make you feel that a demon has taken possession of your body. You may have a fever that feels like the fires of hell, a body that aches like a tin man who hasn't been oiled, nausea so bad you may believe an alien has taken refuge in your stomach, and a congestive headache that feels like your brain is trying to escape through your eyeballs.

Despite these horrors, the flus of yesteryear were actually a lot more serious than those of today. In fact, millions died during the worldwide flu epidemic of 1917–18. Today, the flu's symptoms may be as mild as a low-grade fever with aches and perhaps a slight headache.

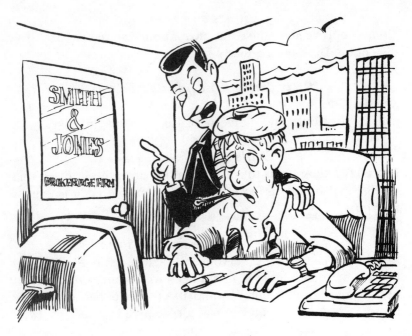

"When it gets to 103, sell."

Schools and worksites are literally flu factories because of the flu's highly contagious nature. The increased risk of getting the flu is but another price we pay for sharing the company of others. Normally it's worth the price, but you may not think so during those seemingly endless days in bed when the flu's hellfire consumes you.

Whatever symptoms you have, flu is no fun, and it's always worthwhile to know of specific strategies that may bring you back to life sooner.

Old stand-bys

Rest, warmth, and fluids are basic to the treatment of the flu. Rest is very helpful, though if you have the energy for simple chores, you should do them, as long as you don't exhaust yourself.

Warmth is primarily a preventive measure to avoid getting a chill. Lots of fluids are very important to avoid dehydration and to help the body eliminate the waste products from infection. If you drink juices, it is best to dilute them half and half with water.

Eat your soup
Eating hot chicken soup has been found to have antiviral effects. A million-jillion mothers couldn't be wrong.

Try vitamin C
Although it is still controversial whether vitamin C is helpful in treating flu, research suggests that it does have some preventive effect. Since it is unlikely that any adverse side effects result from short-term, high doses of vitamin C, it couldn't hurt to try this strategy. Consider taking one gram every four hours during flu symptoms.

Be anti-antibiotics
The flu is caused by a virus, and antibiotics are only helpful for bacterial infection. Since doctors often feel compelled to do something for you and since patients often demand that something be done, antibiotics are occasionally prescribed for the flu even though they won't help.

Get down on aspirin
Aspirin is generally effective in lowering fever and reducing body aches, but it should *never* be used for a person with influenza. Fever is an important defense of the body in its effort to fight infection; by taking aspirin and lowering the fever, you are delaying your healing. Do you really want to do that? If you have a high fever (103 degrees or higher) with much aching and if other strategies are not working rapidly enough, consider taking acetaminophen (Tylenol) for relief. Although it is a drug, it is generally safer to take than aspirin.

Give yourself a sponge bath
A sponge bath can be wonderful, just like your mother may have given you when you could fit in the kitchen sink. Use warm, not hot, water.

An epsom salt bath
Put three tablespoons of Epsom salts in a warm bath and soak in it for twenty minutes.

A spicy treatment
Garlic and cayenne in combination are beneficial herbs for treating infections. Garlic has infection-fighting properties, and cayenne is good for the blood, stimulates the heart, and helps spread the action of the garlic throughout the body. Both of these herbs are available in capsules.

An herbal booster
Echinacea is an herb that stimulates the immune system and has antiviral action. At the first sign of flu, take a dropperful of Echinacea extract, approximately thirty drops in water or tea, once a day for three or four days.

Duck soup?
Oscillococcinum is a homeopathic medicine that is a microdose taken from the liver and heart of a duck. Although this may sound a bit like witchcraft, solid research has shown it to be an effective remedy for the flu. Biologists have discovered that 80 percent of all ducks have every known influenza virus in their digestive tracts. Perhaps the homeopathic dose of the liver and heart also contains helpful antibodies that counter flu. Considering that chicken soup has antiviral properties, it is conceivable that this condensed version of duck soup is similarly therapeutic.

Flu away with homeopathics
Two other homeopathic medicines are often effective for treating the flu, though each is primarily good for a specific pattern of

symptoms. *Gelsemium* (yellow jasmine) *6* or *30* is good when your flu makes you feel tired, weak, and heavy. Your eyelids look heavy and droop. You may have chills and a headache in the back part of your head. You have no thirst and feel great relief after you urinate. When you need *Bryonia* (wild hops), you have body aches, feel irritable, and your pain is aggravated by any type of motion. You may have a headache in the front part of your head and feel you need to lie still because any motion intensifies the pain. A light touch, stooping, eating, or talking aggravate the headache, while firm pressure and lying still relieves it. You feel better in a cool room and are aggravated in a warm room. You have an intense thirst for cool drinks and tend to have a dry, hacking cough. Generally, it is recommended to take the 6th or 30th potency of these medicines, usually four times a day for one to three days, stopping if symptoms abate sooner.

Run away from the flu
Research has shown that exercise temporarily increases your white blood cells, thus helping you to fend off flu viruses. This strategy, however, is better as a preventive measure than as a treatment, since you're usually too exhausted to exercise once the flu bug has struck.

INSOMNIA
▼

Falling asleep can be so easy, and yet at times be so hard. When insomniacs meet with narcoleptics (people who have an uncontrollable tendency to fall asleep throughout the day), each is inevitably jealous of the other's condition.

The solution for people having difficulty falling asleep is to avoid trying so hard. However, telling an insomniac to *not* try to fall asleep is like telling someone who is starving to try to fast when sitting at a dinner table.

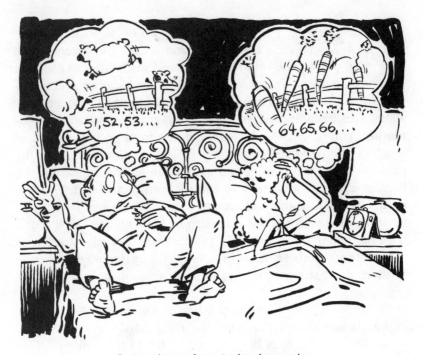

Insomniac and vegetarian insomniac.

It may be reassuring to know that 15 to 25 percent of all adults suffer regularly from insomnia. Somehow, though, this awareness usually doesn't make falling asleep any easier. In fact, there are probably readers who will now stay up nights trying to organize 3:00 A.M. meetings of Insomniacs Anonymous.

While some insomniacs have difficulty falling asleep, others wake frequently and have problems staying asleep. Whichever problem you are experiencing, this is one situation whose solution can't be found by sleeping on it.

The good news is that not everyone necessarily needs eight hours of sleep a night. Some people define themselves as insomniacs because they sleep only five or six hours a night. Actually they should think of themselves as high-energy people who don't need a lot of sleep. Some people's body rhythms are such that their highest and most creative energy period occurs late at night.

The wakeful state that these people experience is not a sign of illness; it may simply be a signal—sometimes an annoyingly loud signal—that the person should use this alert time to do some creative work.

Perhaps the best way to determine if you're getting enough sleep at night is if you feel rested and refreshed upon waking. If you *don't* feel rested and need some help, read the next set of strategies. Soon you may be getting sleepy, very sleepy, very very sleepy . . .

Relaxation trick #1
Hypnotize yourself. Feel total relaxation in your feet, then slowly feel the relaxation move up your body. Tell yourself: I am falling asleep. Use diaphragmatic breathing, which will help relax you further (see Strategy 8 in the Asthma section).

Relaxation trick #2
Massage the soles of your feet, or preferably, have them massaged for you. This can be very relaxing.

Relaxation trick #3
Take a warm bath to which you add a couple of drops of one or more essential oils such as orange blossom, meadowsweet, or hops.

Hops to it
Hops is the herb used to make beer, and it is also used by herbalists to help people go to sleep. Some people brew a tea of it; others purchase the hops leaves and insert them into a pillow. You could also buy a dream pillow; this is a small pillow filled with various sweet-smelling herbs which help you to think sweet thoughts and dream sweet dreams.

Herbal sedatives
Steep one teaspoon each of valerian root, scullcap, and catnip for twenty minutes. One cup will relax the body and calm the mind.

Another good combination of herbs is chamomile, passion flower, and hops. These herbs are available in capsule form too, though drinking a warm tea of them has an additional relaxing effect.

Don't count sheep, count on sheep's wool
Wool blankets are better able to regulate skin and body temperature than synthetic blankets. This comfortable comforter may help you sleep better.

Caffeine and other stimulants lurk in unsuspecting places
Avoid caffeinated products, including colas, aspirin, diet pills, black tea, and, of course, coffee. Nicotine in cigarettes is also a stimulant.

Warm milk rarely works
Despite folklore that has long suggested that warm milk helps people to sleep, research has shown that it is rarely helpful. In fact, non-fat and low-fat milk can actually stimulate the brain's activity.

Avoid cat naps
Day naps should be avoided if you have problems with insomnia. Save your best forty winks for nighttime.

Exercise earlier in the day and avoid it at night
A well-exercised body is less likely to experience insomnia, except when exercise is done within two hours of bedtime. Late-night aerobic activity can generate too much energy to fall asleep easily.

Bedrooms are for sleeping
Avoid using your bedroom for stressful activities such as paying bills or doing work. Let your bedroom be a soothing, quiet, and relaxing place to be at all times.

150

Create a sleep ritual

When it's time for sleep, close the shades, get into your special bed clothes, brush your teeth, turn off the lights, and fluff the pillow. Mentally scan your body and sense where you feel tension. Tighten this place and then relax it. Take a couple of slow, deep breaths. You may also want to make certain that you are getting adequate but not too much ventilation. Do whatever other activities make you feel comfortable, secure, and relaxed.

Unmedicate yourself

Many prescription and over-the-counter drugs, including decongestants and aspirin, can disturb sleep. Talk with your doctor to see if you can reduce the dosage or change the prescription.

Rest assured, sedatives disrupt sleep

Besides being addictive, sedatives disturb deep sleep, leading you to wake unrefreshed. Occasional use of sedatives may be worthwhile, but avoid regular use.

Don't drink your sleep away

Alcohol may make you drowsy, but it disrupts sleep patterns and creates unrefreshing sleep.

Try sex

Making love can be very energizing at times, but it can also be extremely relaxing, thus helping to get the sandman's attention. (Don't try this if it causes anxiety instead.)

Eight hours isn't necessary

Research has suggested that insomniacs actually need less sleep than others. Don't feel pressured to get a full eight hours every night; you may experience less anxiety about yourself and may be able to sleep better, even if you do sleep less.

Coffee as a sedative

Homeopathic doses of coffee (*Coffea*) actually help to relax the mind and body. Take *Coffea 6* or *30* thirty minutes before bedtime and then again as you get into bed. This is particularly effective if you're physically as well as mentally restless.

Sweet dreams with passion flower
Passiflora 3 (passion flower) is perhaps the closest to a generic homeopathic medicine for insomnia in children or the elderly, as well as for those with a hyperactive mind (too many ideas and anxieties crowding in on you).

Take two mantras and call me in the morning
A mantra is usually a one- or two-syllable word that you repeat over and over and over again. You use it as a way to calm the mind, though it can also clear the mind and encourage sleep. You don't have to use Sanskrit words as a mantra; you can use whatever you like: "one," "God," "love," or even "sleep."

Talk out loud
By vocally releasing the things that are bothering you, you are letting go of them. Acknowledge your anxieties, insecurities, and fears out loud. Get these emotions out and they may let you sleep. Keeping a journal can also be very cathartic.

IRRITABLE BOWEL SYNDROME
....▼....................................

Irritable bowel syndrome (IBS), also known as spastic colon, can be painful, anxiety-provoking, just plain uncomfortable, and even disabling. Believe it or not, IBS is the cause of more industrial absenteeism than any other condition, even more than the common cold.

Typically, with IBS you suffer from abdominal pain, bloating, and nausea. You also usually experience diarrhea or constipation (which may alternate).

Despite all of the troubles it brings, IBS doesn't actually involve tissue damage or inflammation in any part of the intestines. Because of this lack of physical manifestation, IBS was considered for many years to be a psychosomatic disorder. This is no longer the case. Although your emotional and mental state may affect this condition, physiological factors also can trigger this syndrome. Some people with IBS experience an exacerbation of symptoms after eating certain foods. Also, research has shown that people with IBS tend to be more sensitive to abdominal gas, leading them to feel greater stomach pains than others.

Here are some strategies to help you and your bowels become less irritable and more friendly.

Find the culprit
Many IBS sufferers are allergic to one or more foods. The most common offenders are wheat, eggs, corn, milk products, peanuts, soy, fish, fruits (especially citrus), raw vegetables, coffee, and tea. Fried and greasy foods also cause problems in some people. Avoid any food or drink you suspect for at least a week and see if you notice any improvement in your health. It is best to eliminate one suspect at a time.

Be a detective
Keep a diary about your life and bowel habits. Pay careful attention to which events, foods, or hormonal changes may be related to your bowel habits. See if you can discover those factors that trigger an attack so that you can possibly prevent future problems.

Graze
Instead of eating three relatively large meals, eat five or six smaller meals throughout the day.

Your heating pad or mine?
Apply a heating pad or hot water bottle to your abdomen during attacks of abdominal pain; its soothing and relaxing effect will diminish the pain.

Fiberize yourself

Eat foods rich in fiber, such as whole grains (especially wheat or oat bran), legumes, and fresh fruits and vegetables. If you're having difficulty digesting such foods, try psyllium husks or one of the fiber products, such as Metamucil.

Don't be artificially sweet

Sorbitol, an artificial sweetener, is known to worsen IBS because it is not easily digested. Some physicians believe that sorbitol isn't the only sweetener that can aggravate IBS. Fructose, mannitol, and other sweeteners may also be a problem because some people cannot absorb these sugars, causing them to ferment in the abdomen (the sugars, not the people).

Cut the fat

Fats increase the muscular contractions of the colon and can irritate an already irritable bowel.

Drink up

Drinking lots of water and other liquids helps to replace the vital fluids lost as a result of diarrhea and helps lubricate the compacted stools when you are constipated. Coffee and tea, however, should be avoided because they can irritate the bowel.

Herbal soothers

Mix one-half ounce of marshmallow root, one-quarter ounce of valerian root or lady's slipper, and one-eighth ounce of slippery elm. Boil this mixture in two pints of water for fifteen minutes. Strain while warm. Drink one-half cup every two hours during the day.

Chill out

Many IBS sufferers appear cool and collected externally, while they hold a great deal of anxiety and anticipation inside. This extra effort can cause extra tension on the bowel. Don't be cool. Express yourself.

Less is more

There are IBS sufferers who try to stay active. It may be better, or at least less stressful, to do fewer activities in a calmer, more relaxed manner.

Say good-bye to your anxieties

One way to do this is to remember a major anxiety that you once thought would never go away. Remember how it did? So will your present anxieties. New ones will inevitably arise, but if you have an underlying attitude that all things must pass, you can be less anxious about your problems and more capable of moving on.

Natural tranquilizers

Yoga and meditation are natural tranquilizers which help to calm you physically, emotionally, and mentally. Try to do twenty to thirty minutes of yoga once a day and twenty minutes of meditation twice a day.

Jog it loose

Jogging and other forms of exercise help to relieve stress and release endorphins, the body's natural painkillers. Also, by improving muscle tone, you may also help improve bowel tone.

MENOPAUSE
▼

*The most creative force in the world
is a menopausal woman with zest.*
Margaret Mead

As one woman friend once said, "Menopause is like a long premenstrual syndrome, and because it's the last one, it's a doozie."
Usually menopause begins when a woman is between forty-

five and fifty-five years of age. Approximately 75 percent of women experience some discomfort just prior to and during menopause, including hot flashes, vaginal dryness, depression, irritability, dizziness, insomnia, and night sweats. These symptoms can recur for one, two, or more years.

The most severe symptoms of menopause are usually treated by conventional physicians with hormone-replacement therapy. Because women are encouraged to take these drugs for the rest of their life and because they can have serious side effects, women and their doctors should use them judiciously and, when possible, seek safer alternatives.

Perhaps the most disturbing aspect of hormone-replacement drugs is the assumption that sometimes underlies their prescription: that the woman is deficient in female hormones. The reduction in female hormones is not a deficiency; it is a natural decrease in the body's ability to become pregnant. Assuming that this is a deficiency state is like assuming that a two-year-old girl is hormone-deficient because her breasts are not developed.

Some physicians assert that the more natural alternatives to hormone-replacement therapy are unproven, and some believe that the alternatives are strange bits of folklore which are closer to quackery than to science. This perspective is ironic since one of the most common hormone-replacement drugs, Premarin, is actually taken from the urine of a pregnant horse.

Rather than call each other strange or weird, now more than ever it seems worthwhile for us to investigate systematically to find safe measures and carefully evaluate when safer or more drastic measures can best be applied. Then, hopefully, this change of life can be a time of joy and personal transformation.

Here are some strategies to help the menopausal woman to maintain or re-attain her zest.

Don't dilate those blood vessels

Large meals, alcohol, coffee, spicy foods, and strong emotions can dilate blood vessels and cause the body to grow warmer. Don't add fuel to the fire of those hot flashes.

156

Fire extinguishers on hot flashes

Take 500 to 1,000 mg. of vitamin C with each meal; it strengthens capillaries and can help regulate body temperature. Vitamin C and vitamin B-complex enhance the effectiveness of estrogen, thus aiding the body to adapt to the reduction of this hormone. Bioflavonoids work synergistically with vitamin C and should be taken with it. Taking 200 IUs of vitamin E and 50 to 100 mcg. of selenium with meals helps heart function and also helps the body better regulate its temperature.

Herbal extinguishers

The following herbal cocktail is great for women with hot flashes: black cohosh, licorice root, sarsaparilla, blessed thistle, false unicorn root, red raspberry leaf, elder, and squaw vine. Mix a couple of tablespoons of this mixture and steep for twenty minutes in hot water. Drink a cup or two a day. Licorice root, elder, and unicorn root contain a substance similar to estrogen, and sarsaparilla contains a substance similar to progesterone. If you have high blood pressure or water retention, don't use the licorice root.

Fan the flames

Perhaps the simplest and quickest way to cool down during a hot flash is to pull out a small, battery-powered electric fan.

Douse the flames

By drinking lots of water, especially after exercising, you help your body regulate its temperature.

Natural clothing

Natural-fiber clothing reduces some of the heat you feel during hot flashes.

A female ginseng

Dong quai is an herb that is considered a female ginseng. This tonifying herb is an overall body-strengthening remedy. It also contains folic acid and B_{12}, which help prevent pernicious anemia.

An herb for the change of life

The Bach Flower Remedy, walnut flower, is helpful during major life changes. Place a couple of drops under the tongue as needed.

Bee yourself

Bee pollen contains both male and female hormones and can be effective in relieving hot flashes and other symptoms of menopause. Take a couple of bee pollen capsules twice a day or at least 500 milligrams.

How dry I am . . . how dry I was

Vaginal dryness is a common symptom of menopausal women. Some simple lubricants can be used, including K-Y jelly, Calendula (marigold) cream, and coconut oil. You can also simply open a vitamin E capsule and use a few drops of the oil. These oils last longer than vegetable oils.

Consistent sex

This more-than-one-minute (hopefully!) healing strategy helps to prevent vaginal dryness and swings in estrogen level. Research has shown that sexual desire does not decrease during menopause and, in fact, actually increases for many women.

The soy of menopause

Soybeans, peas, and cucumbers are rich in natural estrogens; eating them can help alleviate some symptoms of menopause.

Are the side effects worth it?

Estrogen-replacement drugs raise copper levels in the blood and lower zinc levels. Elevated copper can cause moodiness, and zinc deficiency can lead to depression. These symptoms are common problems of menopause, and estrogen drugs augment them. If you are feeling these emotions strongly and are taking these drugs, talk to your doctor. He or she may choose to lower your dose of estrogen or seek safer alternatives.

A healthy dose of family and friends

Research has found that women with restricted social networks (women with little family life or few friends) suffer the most serious symptoms of menopause. Take a dose of family and friends as often as possible.

You're not just getting older, you're evolving

The negative picture of growing older can create additional wrinkles and worry warts, inside and out. Growing older is not the problem; it's the negative baggage carried with it that can weigh you down. Be proud of surviving so long, and think of wrinkles as the merit badges of survival.

May you die young . . . as late in life as possible

Youth is a state of mind, not a specific age parameter. Zest and love of life are ageless and create a radiance that can help you deal with whatever difficulties you are experiencing during this transitional period in your life. If this zest is missing from your life, find it—and enjoy yourself in the search!

NAUSEA AND VOMITING

Tossing your cookies sounds like fun, except when you understand its slang meaning. While not an enjoyable activity, vomiting, throwing up, heaving, or whatever you prefer to call it is a valuable, even lifesaving defense of the body.

Gastric irritation can occur from ingesting poison or harmful bacteria, and nausea and vomiting are the body's forthright efforts to deal with and eliminate this irritation in the quickest way possible. Nausea and vomiting are also the body's response to ingesting too much alcohol, too much food, or even just a little bit of a food which the body cannot efficiently digest. Nausea and vomiting are common for pregnant women during their first

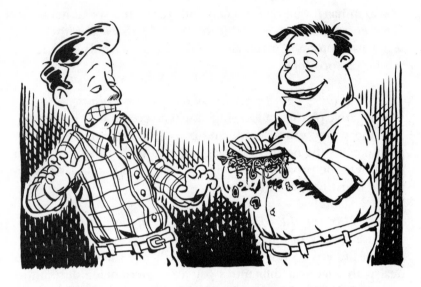

*"It's a peanut butter sandwich with anchovies, okra and
blue cheese in a mustard-garlic-fudge sauce. I'm treating
my nausea with a homeopathic approach."*

trimester. Despite the intense discomfort that morning sickness
causes for pregnant women, the good news is that women who
experience it also secrete higher amounts of hormones that reduce the chances of miscarriage or stillbirth. The body's efforts
to protect itself are at work again.

The word nausea is derived from the Greek word for "ship."
Nausea caused by seasickness and other forms of motion sickness
seems to be an inherent response of the body to certain forms
of disequilibrium. Vomiting and nausea are also common for virtually anyone who is stressed in any way that makes you sick.
Horror movies, disgusting sights, and cruel behavior can all lead
to disequilibrium and gastric disturbances. Most people who feel
nauseous have little or no appetite, which is another helpful
defense of the body. Here are some strategies that may help you.

Don't add fuel to the fire
Try fasting. If you have an appetite, eat lightly; try such things as vegetable soup (the best choice), rice and steamed vegetables, toast, or grated apples. Avoid fats.

Keep liquidated
Avoid dehydration from vomiting, especially if you have diarrhea at the same time. Drink vegetable broth, rice water (the excess water from cooking rice—this is great for nausea), carbonated water, ginger ale, or chamomile or ginger tea (grate one teaspoon of fresh ginger and make tea with it). Drink in sips, not in gulps. Suck on ice chips if nothing else will stay down. Avoid coffee and black tea, which can irritate your stomach.

Culture yourself
Miso soup (made from fermented soy beans and /or other grains) can be made in a minute and contains friendly bacteria which help you digest your food more efficiently. Yogurt also has these friendly bacteria; it's best to eat the unflavored kind.

Compress yourself
Apply hot and cold compresses to the abdomen. Apply hot compresses for three minutes and then cold compresses for one minute. Repeat this after thirty minutes.

Take a breather
Diaphragmatic breathing (as described in the Asthma section) is wonderfully relaxing and helps your body recharge itself.

Morning sickness vitamins
Some clinicians recommend taking up to 50 mg. of vitamin B_6 and 25 mg. of zinc per day to combat nausea from pregnancy.

Ipecac for nausea?
Ipecac is widely known as a substance which induces nausea and vomiting, and because of this, it is a common homeopathic med-

icine for treating such symptoms when given in very small doses. It is particularly helpful when you have acute, persistent nausea and do not feel relieved after vomiting. You usually have little thirst and are nauseous at the smell of food. You often have increased salivation and a clean (not coated) tongue. *Ipecac 6* or *30* can be taken every other hour for a day.

Spell relief: h-o-m-e-o-p-a-t-h-y

Another helpful homeopathic medicine is *Pulsatilla* (wind-flower). It is most useful when you experience nausea or vomiting after eating rich or fatty foods, especially ice cream. You tend to feel worse in warm rooms and feel better in a cool one. *Pulsatilla 6* or *30* is recommended every three hours for a day. *Nux vomica* (poison nut) is commonly used for nausea or vomiting from mental exertion, overeating, or from the use of alcohol, coffee, or drugs (therapeutic or recreational). It is for people who tend to be irritable and constipated. Take *Nux vomica 6* or *30* every three hours for a day.

OSTEOPOROSIS
▼

Both bones and eggshells are made primarily of calcium. Although bones can be impressively strong, depending upon their density, they can break like eggshells.

Osteoporosis, a common condition of the elderly, affects women more than men because they have less bone mass and because they produce less estrogen after menopause, which re-duces the body's ability to keep calcium in the bones. Osteo-porosis leads to degeneration of the spine, humpback, and fragile bones—which are more easily fractured. This condition is cre-ating an elderly population which is fragile, weak, and, like an eggshell, breakable.

Osteoporosis is also creating a legion of shorter elderly people

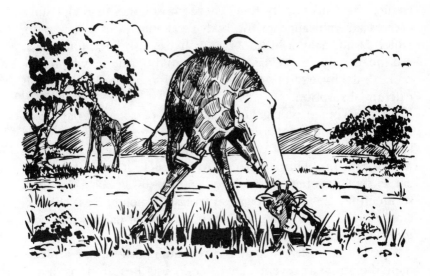

Worst case scenario: Giraffe osteoporosis.

whose vertebrae are compressing against each other due to the loss of calcium from the bone. This epidemic of osteoporosis has created a major market for calcium supplementation. If calcium supplements were listed on the stock exchange, their price would have skyrocketed in recent years. However, if people knew the research about calcium that follows here, the stock's value would have fallen as fast as it rose.

There are numerous countries that have a very low rate of osteoporosis even though their population consumes as little as 200 mg. of calcium a day, considerably less than the 1,000 to 1,500 mg. of calcium that most doctors recommend for pre- and post-menopausal women. The problem in this country is that most women consume too many things that leech the calcium out of their bones.

Research has shown that excessive protein, especially red meat (which contains twenty times more phosphorus than calcium), creates an imbalance in the body's calcium/phosphorus ratio, which is normally a little over 1:1. It has also been found that red meat stimulates release of parathyroid hormone, which promotes calcium excretion. Fats, especially saturated fats, inhibit calcium absorption.

Eskimo women, who get over 2,000 mg. of calcium a day (from their consumption of fish bones), and exercise regularly, are known to have one of the highest rates of osteoporosis in the world. This problem is not due to bad luck. It is because they eat so much protein (as much as 250 to 400 grams a day) and so much fat, this excess causes increased calcium loss. This example highlights the importance of looking at factors that help *and* hinder calcium absorption.

Conventional physicians often recommend hormone-replacement therapy as a preventive to osteoporosis. Research has shown that lifelong use of these hormones helps to maintain bone strength, though it does not restore bone loss that has already occurred. More troubling about the use of these drugs are the numerous studies indicating that they create side effects, including increased chances of endometrial cancer and heart disease. Also, once a woman stops taking these drugs, calcium excretion is significantly increased.

Here are some strategies that are less costly than drugs, both financially and otherwise, and with fewer side effects. Since having adequate calcium levels in the bone is dependent on building bone strength during youth, it is best to take measures to prevent osteoporosis as early in life as possible. Although the best time to start was when you were a child; the second best time is today.

Move your bod

Exercise, especially weight-bearing exercise such as walking, tennis, dancing, rope-jumping, basketball, and backpacking, helps build strong bones. Swimming is not considered a weight-bearing exercise because of the zero-gravity environment of water.

Do kinder, gentler exercises
Free the neck! Power to the pelvis! Liberate the vertebrae 31! Doing yoga and other gentle exercises helps make you limber and stronger. However, headstands and shoulderstands should not be done if you already have osteoporosis.

Calcium-rich foods
Sardines, salmon, green leafy vegetables, broccoli, tofu with calcium sulfate, mineral water, and sesame seeds all will supply your body with calcium. If you choose to get your calcium from milk, yogurt, or cheese, it is recommended to consume low-fat or nonfat products because the body will be better able to assimilate their calcium.

Avoid calcium vampires
Calcium vampires are substances that suck the calcium out of your bones. In other words, they stimulate the body to excrete more calcium than is being put into it. Some of these substances are alcohol, caffeine, salt, animal protein, fats, tobacco, distilled water, oxalic acid-rich foods (chard, rhubarb, spinach, and chocolate), and aluminum (absorbed from baking soda, aluminum pots, and from certain deodorants). Phosphorus-rich foods and drinks also impair calcium absorption, the worst offenders being soda drinks, milk and milk products, and many processed foods.

Avoid calcium vampire drugs
Many drugs disrupt calcium absorption or metabolism, including antacids, antibiotics, anti-depressants, barbiturates, cholesterol-reducing drugs, corticosteroids, diuretics, laxatives, and chemotherapeutic drugs.

Support stomach acid
An inadequate amount of stomach acid can lead to poor absorption of calcium. To increase stomach acid, eat charcoal-barbequed

foods or charcoal supplements, eat more slowly, and don't wash your food down too quickly with a drink.

Go outside
Vitamin D is important for calcium absorption. You can absorb vitamin D by being exposed to the sun. Get a healthy dose of this sun vitamin (when possible, an hour or two per day), but don't overdo it.

Fish for fish oil
Fish oil has a healthy dose of vitamin D, which helps the body absorb calcium.

Do the calcium-magnesium team
Calcium and magnesium are a team that work together in your body, so if you take calcium, you should also take magnesium. Pre-menopausal women should take approximately 1,000 mg. of calcium a day. During menopause, they should take about 1,500 mg. The best calcium supplements (in order of preference) are hydroxyapatite, citrate, lactate, gluconate, and carbonate. It is best to avoid taking large doses of calcium at one time; better to take smaller doses more frequently. Also, don't think that mega-doses of calcium are better than the above recommendations; too much calcium can create problems because it displaces iron, manganese, and zinc, and it can lead to kidney stones. The dose of magnesium should be at least 50 percent of the dose of calcium. For additional help, take 1,000 mg. of vitamin C, which helps to create collagenous fibers to which the calcium of the bone is attached.

Supplemental supplements
Boron, zinc, copper, and manganese are essential for bone integrity. They are all in green leafy vegetables. Boron is of special value; it has been found to stimulate higher estrogen levels and increase bone density. Supplementation of 5 mg. per day is recommended.

Horsetail tea
It won't grow you a tail, but this herb is rich in calcium and silica and can help build strong bones.

Be born black
While this is not a one-minute strategy, evidence does show that black people do not experience as much osteoporosis as white people, possibly because they have greater bone mass.

PAIN

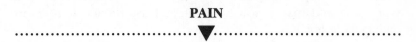

The great engineer of the universe has made man as perfectly as he could make him, and he could not have invented a better device for his maintenance than to provide him with a sense of pain.
René Descartes

Pain has been referred to as a temporary condition caused by a deficiency of morphine. Actually, this isn't too far from the truth, since the body does create its own opiate-like substances called endorphins which deaden pain. Luckily, you can't get arrested for carrying opiate-derivatives in your brain.

Pain is a very subjective feeling. The International Association for the Study of Pain defines pain as an unpleasant sensory or emotional experience associated with actual or potential tissue damage. Whatever the source or nature of the pain, it is calling, even demanding, your attention. Pain is an inherent protection device that nature has given us. It is sometimes difficult to acknowledge the value of pain when you experience its wrath. Still, pain is absolutely essential for the survival of the human species. Among other benefits, it encourages us to learn from our mistakes and to avoid potentially dangerous experiences. To try to understand what it is saying is worthwhile, though not always easy.

The most common chronic pain syndromes are backache, headache, joint pain, and pain from injury. Pain itself is not a disease but a symptom of disease or injury. Simply treating the pain doesn't necessarily change the condition, and this is why painkillers offer only short-term relief at best.

Conventional medical treatment for pain usually consists of medication, nerve blocks, and surgery. Although these approaches may provide certain benefits, they encourage you to be passive, giving you a sense that you don't have much control over your own pain or your own life.

The following strategies will help you take greater control of your pain and may eradicate it or at least reduce it to more manageable levels.

Breathe into the pain
Resisting pain can sometimes aggravate it, just like trying to untie a knot by pulling it tighter. Taking a deep, abdominal breath into and through the pain can be relaxing and healing. Focus your attention on the pain and imagine you are inhaling and exhaling through the primary site of the pain. Breathing into the pain while doing yoga exercises can provide additional therapeutic effects.

Get in hot water
Sitting in a hot tub can be wonderfully therapeutic.

Get tense
Tightening the area around the pain for a couple of seconds and then releasing it is a good trick to reduce the pain.

Get to the point
There are acupressure points all over your body that can be effective in reducing the pain and beginning healing. The best points are never immediately on the primary source of the pain. Seek out *trigger points*, that is, points that seem hypersensitive to the touch. Sometimes good points are around joints that are near the pain; sometimes they are on the other side of the body

parallel to where the pain is. Press the point firmly with your thumb for five seconds, release, and then repeat the pressure several times.

Get it handed to you

Ask a friend to practice laying on of hands, which is an ancient healing practice that has been used in numerous cultures and is used today by thousands of nurses and other health professionals in hospitals. The person doing it should concentrate, imagining loving and healing energies emitting from his hands into your body. He may choose to hold his hands near the area of pain, though you should encourage him to use intuition to determine where to apply the energy. While your friend is there, perhaps he can also give you a massage, which can be wonderfully relaxing and pain-relieving.

Have a spicy life

Eat chili peppers. They contain capsaicin, which has been found to stimulate secretion of endorphins and reduce the release of a neurotransmitter, substance P, which short-circuits the perception of pain.

Natural aspirin

A primary ingredient of aspirin is derived from willow bark. Make a tea using it.

Dear Diary

Keep a pain journal. By observing carefully when and where you experience pain, you can sometimes find certain patterns to it, and then try to break these patterns. You may, for instance, discover that you develop your symptoms when you do not get enough sleep, do inadequate physical exercise, miss a meal, eat certain foods, or visit relatives.

Describe and draw the pain

Describe the pain in as much detail as possible including shape and color; then draw it with crayons or colored pens or pencils.

Imagine and draw the shapes and colors you feel may soothe it; then visualize these colors and shapes in your body.

Mental technology

Research on biofeedback has not only shown its value in teaching people to relax but also its influence on many bodily functions. Biofeedback is very valuable in teaching people to have greater control and direction over their bodies and thus over their pain. Learn how to use it.

Meditation technology

Meditation not only helps you achieve greater relaxation, it encourages more focused concentration, giving you greater control of your mind, and thus greater control over your sense of pain.

Hypnotize yourself

Auto-hypnosis is a popular technique for relaxation and can be used effectively for healing and pain control. One hypnosis strategy, called glove anesthesia, is to put yourself in a trance and imagine your hand to be numb, heavy, and wooden. Then, move your hand to the part or parts of the body that feel pain and imagine those parts feeling similarly relaxed, heavy, and numb.

Stimulate those endorphins

Research has found that exercise increases endorphin levels in the blood. The increase in these opiate-like substances is one reason that athletes sometimes feel high when they are exercising. Likewise, exercise may help reduce your pain. However, this strategy should not be considered if the exercise *causes* pain.

Massage the sole

Your feet, especially their soles, have thousands of nerve endings. By massaging them, you are stimulating various parts of the body that the nerves feed, thus reducing pain. The joy and relaxation that massaging the feet creates is good for the sole and for the soul.

170

Believe in belief
Whatever you do to relieve your pain, believe in it and it will work better. Research has shown that approximately 33 percent of people with pain experience relief of symptoms from a placebo.

Distract yourself
Try not to let pain interfere with your life. Keep busy with activities that require concentration so that you can forget about your pain for a while.

Misery loves company
Consider joining a support group of people who experience chronic pain. It's best to avoid groups which simply complain about their problems; instead, seek out a group that shares information about strategies that are helpful in dealing with pain.

Empower yourself
A sense of control over your life is therapeutic in itself. The decision to utilize strategies to help yourself may be almost as helpful as actually doing them.

PREMENSTRUAL SYNDROME
▼

Approximately 50 percent of all women experience various physical and /or psychological symptoms prior to their menstruation. Some experience quite mild symptoms, while others can have reactions dramatic enough to turn Dr. Jekyll into Ms. Hyde.

In the not too distant past physicians commonly believed that the various troubles women claimed to experience prior to their menstruation were all in their head. It is a relief that physicians finally recognize a physiological aspect of premenstrual syndrome, though simply recognizing a condition as valid is not enough to cure it.

Some physicians theorize that PMS results from a drop in progesterone, sometimes called the "tranquility hormone." Others think that soaring estrogen levels lead to irritable and anxious states. Still others believe that the body's awareness that conception did not occur depresses women physically and psychologically. Whatever the cause, women commonly experience a variety of symptoms from the biological changes occurring in their body, including cramps, breast swelling and tenderness, water retention, moodiness, irritability, headache, backache, insomnia, fatigue, constipation, complexion problems, and food cravings.

The premenstrual state, however, does offer some positive effects. Many women experience greater ability to concentrate, more creativity, and more assertiveness during this period. It is a time to clean and order their home and life. Some women who feel more emotional during this special time cherish these feelings and honor them as an integral part of who they are.

My own wife wears some special jewelry during her premenstrual period, both to remind her of her altered state and to inform me. This one-minute strategy helps us both be aware of this more sensitive phase so that Dr. Jekyll and Ms. Hyde are more self-conscious, empathetic, and friendly to each other.

Here are some others.

A *low-fat diet reduces weight* and PMS
Several studies have indicated that women who eat a low-fat diet have less breast swelling and fewer uncomfortable symptoms during their premenstrual period.

Exercise and leave PMS in the dust
Regular exercise has been found to reduce PMS. Besides increasing the brain's secretion of natural painkilling endorphins, exercise helps to tone and relax muscles, improve circulation, and reduce water retention.

Avoid the PMS aggravators
The following substances can aggravate PMS: coffee (even decaffeinated coffee), black tea, chocolate, colas, salt, dairy products, fats, and alcohol.

Keep track of yourself
Keep a diary and watch for habits or patterns in your life which seem to aggravate your condition. You may discover that certain foods, stresses, emotional states, birth-control pill dosages, or amounts of exercise aggravate or reduce your symptoms.

Oil yourself
Evening primrose oil and vegetable oils (safflower, corn, sunflower, and canola) have gamma-linoleic acid in them, which plays an essential role in creating a natural hormone called prostaglandin, which can relieve premenstrual symptoms. It is recommended to take 200 mg. of evening primrose oil for the ten days preceding your menstrual flow. As for the other oils, consider using them (especially canola) when cooking.

Supplementary, my dear Ms. Watson
About two days before you expect to begin your PMS, take calcium up to 400 mg., magnesium up to 800 mg., vitamin A up to 10,000 IU, vitamin D up to 600 IU, and B-complex (especially B_6) with 50 to 100 mg. of the major components. The B vitamins have calming effects on a woman's emotional state, calcium and magnesium are natural tranquilizers, and several of the other vitamins help the body absorb and make use of these minerals. Remember, do not take large doses of these vitamins all at once; the body is best able to absorb smaller doses taken more frequently, and preferably with meals.

Herbal calcium
Comfrey root, horsetail, oat straw, and lobelia, either in pill form or in a tea, are highly recommended. These herbs can be taken together or individually.

Don't cramp your style

Here are some great herbs to reduce the pain and discomfort of menstrual cramps: black cohosh root, false unicorn root, squaw-vine, blessed thistle, lobelia, pennyroyal, and red raspberry. This combination of herbs doesn't taste great, but wouldn't you rather drink something that doesn't taste good than have cramps that don't make you feel good? Drink a couple of cups of this tea throughout the day. A more simplified version of this concoction is black cohosh root and red raspberry. For those who wish to avoid bad-tasting tea, blend these herbs into a powder and put them in a capsule. Take one to three caps a day, as needed, and don't drink any caffeinated beverages the same day.

More herbs to de-cramp your style

Chamomile and peppermint are both wonderfully soothing herbs that reduce cramping and improve digestion. Make a tea of one or the other, for they work best when they are not combined.

Yogis don't get PMS

Or, at least, they don't get it very badly. A survey of 848 women who practice yoga showed that 77 percent of them experienced reduced symptoms of PMS from doing yoga. The corpse pose is great for relaxing and is best done during the early stages of PMS. The corpse pose is done just as it sounds: lay flat on your back with your legs and arms slightly spread, melt into the floor, and feel relaxation spread over your body. Another good yogic posture is the forward bend, which can be done by sitting on the floor with your legs together straight out in front of you, bending your upper torso so that you can touch your toes—or at least your ankles. Try to hold the forward bend as long as you can do so comfortably; continue to breathe slowly and deeply.

The hot and cold treatment

Hot and cold packs on the abdominal area and lower back can be helpful. The hot application should be used for three minutes, and the cold application for one minute. Repeat this two to four times.

Hot stuff
Take a hot bath, drink hot tea, and apply a hot pad to your abdomen (though not necessarily all at the same time).

Super acupressure
This acupressure treatment for relieving menstrual cramps doesn't use your thumbs but your fists. Place them in your lower back while you lie down. To help you apply firmer pressure, lie on your back on the floor with your feet on a chair or couch. You can also use tennis balls.

Get touched
Ask a friend or spouse to massage your back, abdomen, head, neck, and anywhere that it feels good. Massage will relax you as well as help you feel better.

A sexy strategy
Have sex. It is uncertain if orgasms have a direct effect on relieving cramps or if they simply take your mind off the pain— but who cares as long as it works?

Sleep on it
Get plenty of sleep. It not only relaxes but invigorates you, too.

Homeopathic relief
Magnesia phosphorica (phosphate of magnesium) is indicated when menstrual cramps are relieved by warmth and doubling-up. *Colocynthis* (bitter cucumber) is helpful when the menstrual pains almost force you to double-up, or when you feel terribly irritable. *Chamomilla* (chamomile) is useful for the most severe, unbearable cramping pains and when you are extremely irritable. Whatever medicine fits your symptoms, take it in the 6 or 30

potency every three hours during the discomfort. Stop when the pain stops.

A dab for the emotions too

Homeopathic doses of *Pulsatilla* and *Ignatia* are wonderfully effective for the emotional swings of PMS. *Pulsatilla 6* or *30* is particularly helpful for the weepy, moody, and self-pitying PMS woman, while *Ignatia 6* or *30* is indicated for the irritable, mis-understood, and brooding PMS woman.

Get pregnant

Of course, this strategy is only temporarily effective, and may have its own time-consuming side effects.

Get pregnant II

New research indicates that women who have had a child ex-perience less pain during their menstrual cycle than women who have never given birth.

SINUSITIS
▼

The next time someone tells you that you have a hole in your head, just admit that you do. We all do. In fact, there are eight holes in the skull. Commonly called sinuses, these cavities play an important role in respiration. If we didn't have cavities, just solid bone, our neck probably couldn't support the weight of this top-heavy condition.

Inflammation in these sinuses, called sinusitis, creates head pain, facial tenderness, aching eyes, and even a sensation that feels like the teeth are too long. These symptoms make sinusitis sound like a type of torture, as any sufferer will confirm.

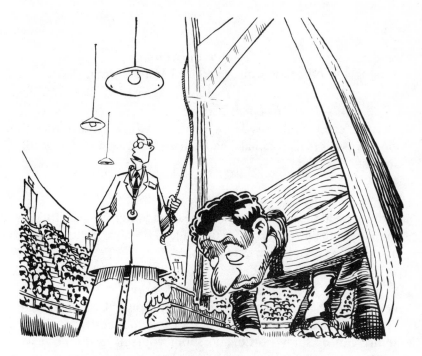

*A professor at the Marie Antoinette School of Medicine
teaches the most effective treatment for sinusitis.*

Sinusitis is most often the revenge of a lingering cold or allergy, which can impede proper nasal drainage. This congestion becomes a breeding ground for infection which then causes the lining in the sinuses to become inflamed and swollen. Other problems that can create congestion leading to sinusitis are polyps, a deviated septum, large or inflamed adenoids, an abscessed or inflamed tooth, or a change in air pressure from flying or swimming.

Sinusitis can create its own revenge too. Unless it is successfully treated, it can sometimes lead to ear infections, bronchitis, or pneumonia.

Although sinusitis sufferers may feel like hiring a plumber to unplug their nose and drain their head, these other strategies should be tried first.

Jog it out of you
Jogging and other vigorous exercise can help drain sinuses.

Alcohol will swell your head
Alcohol causes increased vasodilation, which means that the blood vessels in the cranial area swell and lead to more congestion and inflammation.

Head to the ocean
Swimming in or even being near the ocean offers wonderful relief to many sinusitis sufferers. Avoid valleys because pollen tends to live there and can aggravate sinusitis.

A salt water nasal spray
Perhaps the best nasal spray (and the cheapest) is salt and water. Place a quarter teaspoon of salt and four ounces of water in a squirt gun or spray bottle, and shoot yourself in the nose with it. The salt and water combined will help break up nasal congestion. Blow your nose gently afterward.

Get steamed
Inhaling steam can feel great. Either drape a towel over your head and stand over a pot of boiling water, or take a hot steam shower. For added therapeutic action, add eucalyptus leaves or eucalyptus oil to the boiling water.

Get hot and cold
Alternate hot and cold compresses and place them over the cheekbones and nostrils. Tip your head slightly forward to encourage better drainage through the nose.

Impress yourself
Firm pressure in a circular motion on acupressure points under the eyebrows, on the cheekbones, and at the temples can work wonders.

The massage is the message

Massaging the neck, shoulders, and skull may or may not cure you, but will feel great. Because there are so many nerve endings in your feet, especially on the bottoms, massaging them can sometimes soothe the nervous system and relax the entire body. According to the foot massage system of reflexology, massaging the tips of the toes can be particularly helpful to people with sinusitis.

Don't get smoked

Exposure to cigarette smoke, even second-hand smoke, can be very irritating to the sinuses. Some people will be irritated by a barbeque or by smog. Avoid these irritants whenever possible.

Drink up

Drink lots of fluids (except alcohol) to keep the mucus flowing.

Chicken soup to the rescue, again

Hot chicken soup has been found to stimulate mucus drainage.

Don't blow your brains out

When you blow your nose, do it gently. Blowing too strongly can force the infected mucus back into the sinuses. If, when you blow your nose it sounds like a wildlife mating call, you are blowing too hard.

A sound idea

Relief is sometimes attained by making a repetitious sound. Experiment with various sounds such as "ahhhhhh," "eeeeeee," "ommmmmm," or whatever other sound works for you. Additional benefits are possible if you close your eyes and relax while you say these sounds.

Avoid dry heat

If the heating system in your house or office is providing heat that is too dry, use a humidifer to moisten the air. Check the humidifer regularly for the growth of mold or mildew. If you use an air conditioner, make certain its filter is kept clean.

Head to the spices
Chili peppers, garlic, and horseradish encourage mucus secretion. Add them to meals whenever possible, or simply take capsules of them.

Avoid antihistamines
Although these drugs reduce nasal swelling, they also dry the mucous membranes and therefore encourage greater congestion. It is better to use strategies that stimulate drainage, not stifle it.

Avoid decongestants
Decongestants paralyze the nose hairs (cilia), thus inhibiting the drainage of fluids. They also cause *rebound congestion*, a temporary relief of congestion that is only followed by an increase in it. You may also develop a tolerance to this drug and need stronger and stronger doses of it for it to be effective. Avoid nasal sprays too.

Avoid pool swimming
If you swim, wear a nose plug to prevent chlorinated water from further irritating the sinuses.

Stay grounded
If possible, avoid flying or activities that take you to high altitudes; these can aggravate a sinus condition.

Homeopathic help
Kali bic 6 or 30 is an effective homeopathic medicine for sinus pain at the root of the nose, especially when the person's nasal discharge is thick and stringy. *Pulsatilla 6 or 30* is more commonly given to women or children with sinus problems, espe-

cially when their symptoms are worse at night, or from a warm room, or stooping. People who need *Pulsatilla* may have digestive symptoms that accompany the sinus pains.

SORE THROAT

▼

The throat takes a lot of abuse. It is subjected to bacterial and viral infection, to various airborne irritants such as dust, smoke, and fumes, and to vocal use (and use and use). Considering all the food that we shove down our throat, often with minimal chewing, it's amazing that our throat still speaks to us.

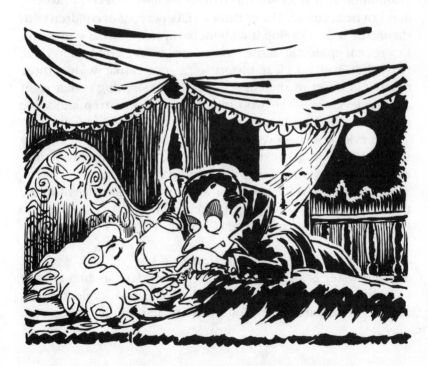

A little known fact: Health-conscious Dracula tests his victims for strep throat before biting them.

Like so many other parts of the body, the throat is quite durable. And yet, it does have its limits. It leaves us speechless or chokes us up with emotion. It gives us a lump in the throat or a pain in the neck. It gets rough with us or can even make it difficult for us to swallow all these metaphors.

Viruses and bacteria may cause a sore throat, but so can open-mouth breathing, artificially heated air, vocal overuse, and anything that creates a dry throat. Streptococcus are the most common bacteria to cause a sore throat. Most physicians recommend taking an antibiotic for such infections, not necessarily for the throat pain but primarily to prevent the possibility of rheumatic fever, a life-threatening condition that is thought to result from the strep traveling to and infecting the heart. The commonly held assumption that links strep throat to rheumatic fever, however, may not be accurate. Thirty-three to fifty percent of children with rheumatic fever develop it without having sore throat symptoms. In a recent epidemic of rheumatic fever among children in Utah, two-thirds had no clear history of a sore throat within three months of onset of rheumatic fever. More startling is that eight of the eleven children who tested positive for strep and were thus prescribed antibiotics still developed rheumatic fever.

This evidence suggests that sore throats may not be related to rheumatic fever, and even if they are, it is questionable if antibiotics can prevent this life-threatening condition.

Rather than attacking strep or any other infective agent in the throat, it may be more appropriate and more effective to stimulate the body's own defenses. The following strategies will help.

Gargle treatment #1

Salt and water is a classic gargle treatment. Mix about a quarter teaspoon of salt with a quarter cup of water and gargle. Use this and the other gargles that follow as often as you feel necessary.

Gargle treatment #2

Sage or mullein tea may be healing to sore throats. Steep one teaspoon of the herb in a cup of water. Gargle for at least ten seconds with three different mouthfuls of tea.

Gargle treatment #3

Place five to ten drops of a tincture of myrrh into a cup of warm water and gargle with it. People have used myrrh since Biblical times, and it is known today to have antiseptic and astringent effects.

Gargle treatment #4

Take the leftover water from cooked barley and add lemon to it for a helpful gargle.

Gargle treatment #5

For stubborn sore throats, take a cotton swab and thoroughly coat the back of the throat with the oil of bitter orange. Expect to gag a little from this, but it will be worth it.

Herbal antibiotics

Garlic and echinacea are probably the most effective herbs for treating infections, so if your sore throat is the result of infection rather than throat irritation, this treatment should be tried. These herbs are available in capsule form. Take a couple of capsules of each three times a day.

An herbal soother

Slippery elm tablets are an old, tried-and-true remedy for sore throat. Their soothing qualities protect mucous membranes in a dry and burning throat. People who can stand the funny taste and strange consistency of slippery elm bark tea should make a brew. Improve the taste with honey and lemon.

Vaporize yourself
Steam inhalation can be helpful, especially if you add herbs such as sage, thyme, or mullein to the water. Stand over this boiling brew with a towel over your head.

A vitamin C lozenge
Suck a 250 to 500 mg. tablet of vitamin C slowly so that its acidic nature can burn out the infection.

Zinc lozenges
Zinc lozenges are often effective for sore throats and colds.

First stage homeopathic
Aconite (monkshood) *6* or *30* is recommended for the first stage of a throat infection. It is particularly good when you have a dry throat and a dry cough, especially when you have developed it after exposure to cold, dry winds. Take it every other hour for a day. If your symptoms do not abate after a single night's rest, consider another homeopathic medicine or strategy.

Bee venom homeopathic
If you have the type of sore throat where there is burning or stinging pains with much swelling, relieved by sucking on an ice cube or drinking cold fluids, take *Apis* (crushed bee) *6* or *30*. Because bee venom is known to cause these burning and stinging pains, homeopathic doses of bee venom can initiate a healing response to these pains. Take it three to six times a day, depending on the intensity of the symptoms. If you seem to need to take it for more than two days, it isn't the correct medicine.

For those scarlet throats
If your symptoms include scarlet red tonsils, or reddened face and lips, with a fever, then *Belladonna* (deadly nightshade) *6* or *30* is the homeopathic medicine for you. Take it three to six times a day, depending on the intensity of your discomfort. If it doesn't work within forty-eight hours, consider another strategy.

That fishbone feeling

If you have one of those sore throats that feels like a fishbone is stuck in there, consider taking *Hepar sulphur* (calcium sulphide) 6 or *30*. This homeopathic medicine is particularly effective when you feel relieved by warm drinks and irritated by cold ones. You might commonly feel chilly and easily aggravated by cold air.

Drugs can dry you out

Various prescription and over-the-counter drugs can dry out your throat and then lead to laryngitis or a sore throat. Check with your doctor to see if the drugs should be changed or reduced.

Throw your toothbrush away!

Using and reusing an old toothbrush may reinfect you. Researchers have estimated that toothbrushes carry more than a million bacteria. A thorough rinsing of the brush is thought to reduce this number only by one half, so it may be prudent to throw away your toothbrush after throat and respiratory infections, and to replace it regularly—at least every three months.

ULCERS

▼

There once was an ulcer from Ulster,
'Twas in a youngster, not oldster,
From stress it arose,
And at times it would doze,
That ulcer had a mind of its ownster.

The average adult has thirty-five million digestive glands. These glands produce one of the most powerful corrosives known—gastric acid. Gastric acid is so strong that it can dissolve a razor blade in less than a week. As a result of this strong acid, the body must create a new stomach lining every three days.

Research has now confirmed that most people with ulcers actually have a normal amount of gastric acid. That's because the problem isn't having too much acid; it's in the body's ability to keep the lining of the stomach intact.

Actually, stomach acid isn't the bad guy. Stomach acid is not only essential for digesting foods, it is vital for our survival because it kills fungi, bacteria, and viruses that are ingested with food. If we didn't have the protection that the gastric acid gives us, we would be more susceptible to food poisoning, parasites, and other digestive dilemmas—including ulcers.

The initial symptoms of an ulcer are usually belching and bloating, which can mislead the sufferer to think that you are just experiencing gas. You may also feel hunger pangs and a burning, gnawing, or sharp pain in the abdominal area. The pains tend to be felt forty-five to sixty minutes after eating a meal, although they can also be experienced on an empty stomach. The pains tend to be temporarily relieved by eating food.

Not too long ago, the most common advice that doctors gave ulcer patients was to eat a bland diet, usually boiled fish, rice, steamed vegetables, and milk: no spices, pizza, chili, and no Mexican, Italian, Indian, or Thai food. (Bummer!) As it turns out, this wasn't such good advice, as there is no real evidence that spicy foods cause or exacerbate ulcers. (Whew!)

There are, however, certain foods, drinks, and behaviors that can increase gastric acids and thus create a problem for those people who are not adequately replacing their stomach lining every three days. Here are some ulcer do's and don'ts:

Milk burns!

Although milk initially coats the stomach walls, providing temporary relief, the stomach secretes increased acid to digest the milk, ultimately making stomach discomforts worse than before. Avoid this rebound effect by avoiding milk.

Painkillers can be stomach killers
Aspirin is known to cause increased bleeding in the stomach, which can exacerbate an ulcer. By the way, some antacids (notably Alka-Seltzer) contain aspirin, so be careful of which antacid you take. Even worse than aspirin are nonsteroidal anti-inflammatory drugs like Motrin or Advil which can irritate the stomach lining and aggravate an ulcer.

Eat smaller meals
Eating smaller meals more frequently is less stressful on your digestive system than eating two or three larger meals. Chew every bite thoroughly.

Pump iron, but don't ingest it
Don't take iron supplements; they can irritate the stomach.

Supplement your stomach lining
Vitamins A, B_6, E, and folic acid help maintain and repair the stomach lining. Zinc can also be helpful.

Ulcer accomplices
Smoking, alcohol, and caffeine don't cause ulcers, but they do reduce the stomach's ability to protect itself, thus increasing the chances that you'll get an ulcer.

An ulcer's friends
Fried foods, citrus fruits, chocolate, alcohol, black tea, and coffee (regular and decaffeinated) increase gastric acids and can aggravate your ulcer.

Fiberize
Fiber can be helpful because it helps to coat and soothe the stomach lining, but avoid foods that have abrasive roughage, such as nuts, seeds, and popcorn.

A cabbage patch will patch your stomach

Cabbage juice is high in L-glutamine, an amino acid that stimulates the secretion of mucus from the stomach's lining. More than just a folk medicine, cabbage juice has been proven to be effective in treating ulcers. Drink juice only from fresh green cabbage. If this is unavailable where you are, you can use celery juice, which also has ulcer-healing compounds.

Appeal to bananas

Unripe plantain bananas, an old folk remedy for ulcers, can now be obtained in dried-extract pill form. These bananas contain a substance which is known to stimulate mucus from the stomach lining, providing a sturdier barrier against gastric acids.

Lick an ulcer with licorice root

Licorice root has been used for centuries in herbal medicine for various conditions, including ulcers. Its protective effects on the stomach lining reduce stomach discomfort. You can get it from an herb or health-food store; you can suck on it, or make a tea from it. If you have high blood pressure though, you should be careful with this herb; it can elevate blood pressure. If this is the case, you should try a new product, deglycyrrhizinated licorice, which eliminates this potential problem; it is available in health-food stores.

A *slippery soother*

Slippery elm is one of the most effective herbs in botanical medicine for soothing inflamed mucous membranes or ulcers. Pour
boiling water over slippery elm powder and let it steep for ten
minutes. Make certain to stir occasionally so that the "Nestle's
Quick Effect" (the undissolved powder settling to the bottom of
the glass) does not occur. Sip.

An *Indian spice is nice*

Turmeric, a popular Indian spice, has been found to protect the
stomach lining due to its powerful antioxidant effects. Consider
adding it to whatever food you cook, though expect its yellow-
orangish nature to turn your food this color.

An *ulcer extinguisher*

Aloe vera is known to be very effective in treating burns, and
can likewise put out the fire of an ulcer. If you have a fresh aloe
plant, open one of the stalks of the plant and spoon out the watery
gel, blend it with water and drink it. If you don't have a plant,
get aloe vera juice from a health food store. (Make certain that
the juice you purchase is digestible; health-food stores sell many
nonedible cosmetics made with aloe vera.)

The *seaweed treatment*

Nori, the type of seaweed in which sushi is usually wrapped, has
an anti-ulcer substance in it. It also has antimicrobial action
against many disease-causing bacteria. You can eat it with sushi,
or simply take the sheets of nori, dampen and cut them, and add
to salads, steamed vegetables, or grain dishes.

Relief is a breath away

Relax, take a couple of deep breaths, relax more deeply; take a
couple more deep breaths, and relax more deeply.

De-stress yourself

Although there is presently insufficient evidence to prove that
stress *causes* ulcers, it is known that if you already have an ulcer,

stress can make it worse. Actually, it isn't the stress that's the problem; it's your response to the stress that can aggravate an ulcer. Do whatever is necessary to both reduce the amount of stress you are experiencing and to learn to deal with it more effectively.

Slow down
Walk and drive more slowly, eat and drink more slowly, and respond to phone calls and doorbells more slowly. You'll still get there, feel better, and may even enjoy everything a little bit more.

Express yourself
Pent-up feelings, especially anger, can irritate you psychologically and physically. Express what you are feeling. If your feelings cannot be expressed in words, go to a place where you won't disturb others and scream. Screaming in your car or into a pillow are probably the two most practical ways to do it.

VAGINITIS
····································▼····································

Scratching an itch is one of life's great pleasures, but not every itch can scratched, especially in public. When this itching also burns and is accompanied by discharge, you have an even greater problem. Such is the case with vaginitis.

The vagina is a perfect breeding ground for infection; its moisture and warmth promote the survival of both sperm and germs. Since the vagina is also close to the anus, it is all too easy for bacteria to spread to it.

Vaginitis (inflammation of the vagina) can be caused by various organisms such as a fungus (Candida albicans), a bacteria (Gardnerella), or a protozoan (Trichomonas vaginalis). Candida, or yeast, is the most common cause of vaginal infections. Yeast infections frequently result from the use of antibiotics, which may help kill the bad bacteria, but also knock off the good bacteria that are important in preventing fungal growth.

Vaginitis can also result from stress, poor diet, chemical irritation (from douches, spermicides, or feminine hygiene sprays), not enough lubrication during intercourse, and drugs or hormones that throw the system out of balance.

Not all vaginal discharges indicate vaginitis. Some vaginal discharges are normal—healthy secretions that are an integral part of the body's own self-cleaning and self-healing functions. If, however, the discharge is profuse, smelly, or discolored, you may have vaginitis. Here are some strategies that may help.

Culture yourself
Eating yogurt and douching with it (one-half teaspoon in a little water) is often effective. Use only unsweetened and unflavored yogurt, and when douching, do so just prior to going to sleep. You can also apply the yogurt directly to the outer genital area. As an alternative, Lactobacillus acidophilus tablets can either be eaten or inserted in the vagina to inhibit yeast imbalance.

A vinegar soak
Vinegar can acidify the vagina and make it less hospitable to infection. Douche with it (two tablespoons per pint of water) or take a bath in it (a half cup in a bathtub). Don't repeat this more than once a day.

Herbal strategies
Goldenseal (*Hydrastis*) and barberry (*Berberis*) contain berberine, which has a direct effect on various bacteria. Use in an herbal douche (this is most appropriate for vaginitis caused by a bacteria). Make a tea with one teaspoon of the powder from one or both of these herbs in one quart of water; let the water cool down before you douche with it. Tea tree oil (*Melaleuca alternifolia*) is also effective for various types of vaginitis; bathe the genital area with it.

Don't overdouche yourself

Douching can wash away friendly bacteria and make you more susceptible to infection. Don't do it more than once a day for a week. During non-infected times, it is generally not necessary to douche.

Wonderful garlic

Garlic, the stinking rose, has both antifungal and antibacterial action. There are numerous ways to use this useful herb. Try to eat a clove of it several times a day. For more sociable types, take odorless garlic capsules.

Zinc for yourself

There is some evidence that women with recurrent vaginitis have low zinc levels in their blood. Try taking a zinc supplement (50 mg. a day).

Wipe correctly or get wiped out

When you wipe after using the bathroom, be certain to wipe from front to back. When wiping from back to front you may accidently spread bacteria from the anus into the vagina.

To sex or not to sex

If having sex hurts, don't do it. It's best to avoid intercourse when you're infected. If you really want to have sex, use vegetable oil or some other natural means of lubrication. If you are having recurrent infections, your partner should get himself checked out to make certain that he is not a carrier. In the meantime, he should use a condom.

Haircut therapy

Some women, especially those who live in hot and humid climates, find that cutting their pubic hair shorter lessens vaginal moistness and helps to prevent vaginitis.

Go natural
Sleep without underwear to let your vagina breathe freely. At other times wear loose, natural-fiber clothing, especially cotton underwear. Avoid wearing pantyhose too frequently since they do not allow proper ventilation, and avoid sitting around in a wet bathing suit.

Smell natural
Avoid deodorant tampons or deodorant sanitary napkins, scented douches, scented or dyed toilet paper, bubble baths, and products containing chemicals with which your vagina may come into contact. Some women are also sensitive to certain detergents; if you suspect you may be, change whatever detergent you are using to wash your clothes (purer brands are available in most health-food stores).

Change pads more frequently
Tampons can become ripe for infection once they become stained with blood. Also, some tampons are so absorbent that they interfere with normal vaginal secretions, thus making you more susceptible to infection. Consider using sanitary napkins whenever possible.

Get in hot and cold water
Alternate hot and cold water in a bath. Ten minutes in each is sufficient.

Get purple
Gentian violet is an external application which is often effective in treating yeast infections. It was once a common medicine prescribed by physicians, but because it can stain clothing and bedding it went out of favor, despite its therapeutic value. It is available at many pharmacies.

Don't get too sweet
Although you may love sweets, so does yeast. A higher blood-sugar level results from eating sweets and drinking alcohol. Avoid

them; eat healthy amounts of whole grains, fresh vegetables, and low fat protein instead.

Psyche yourself out

Psychological stress can directly affect hormones and make a woman more susceptible to infection. Any illness is stressful, but if you can relax so that the body can work its own self-healing wonders, you may become healthier sooner. Meditation is a much more effective way to achieve health-promoting states of relaxation than just lying back and watching television. Don't just sit there, relax!

Part III

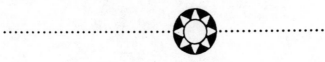

Resources

A NOTE ABOUT USING HOMEOPATHIC MEDICINES

▼

Homeopathic medicines are safe and effective natural remedies for various acute and chronic health problems. There is, however, no single homeopathic medicine that can cure everybody's headache, allergy, flu, or whatever. For the most effective results, these medicines need to be individually prescribed to fit each person's symptoms.

This book provides basic information on common homeopathic remedies for numerous ailments, but it is recommended that you also use one or more of the homeopathic guidebooks mentioned in the bibliography. In addition to offering more detailed information about the homeopathic remedies mentioned in this book, these books will tell you about other homeopathic medicines that may be indicated for treating your unique pattern of symptoms.

Depending on the intensity of the pain, the homeopathic remedies should be taken as often as once every thirty minutes for extreme pain or as little as three times a day when only mild discomfort is felt. Most commonly, people take them every four hours while awake. *or herbals*

Quite distinct from vitamins, homeopathic medicines should not be taken every day or for prolonged periods. People usually do not need to take them for more than two to four days. Most people notice some improvement in health within twenty-four hours. If you do not notice any changes in your symptoms within forty-eight hours, you should consider taking a different homeopathic remedy.

You should not take homeopathic remedies after the pain or discomfort is gone. These medicines—like a spark in lighting a fire—stimulate the body's own healing abilities. Once the fire has been lit, it is not necessary to continue to throw on sparks. In fact, continued dosage of a remedy sometimes results in symptoms like that of an overdose, which vary according to the specific medicine taken. These symptoms will stop shortly after the medicines are no longer taken.

If a homeopathic medicine works temporarily, but the symptoms continue to return over the long run, a deeper-acting homeopathic remedy is probably needed. Professional homeopathic care is recommended in such instances. Homeopaths are trained to prescribe *constitutional medicines*; that is, homeopathic medicines individually chosen to treat the person's totality of symptoms according to that person's genetic disposition, history of acute and chronic illness, and his or her physical and psychological state.

Homeopathic medicines come in different strengths. The most common potencies for the general public are 3, 6, 12, and 30. These numbers refer to the number of times a substance has been diluted and then shaken. Minerals and other substances that are not water soluble are sequentially triturated (ground up) and diluted with a lactose powder. When a substance has been diluted 1:10 (one part of the substance to ten parts distilled water), there is an *x* after the number (*x* in Roman numerals stands for 10). Likewise, when a substance has been diluted 1:100, there is a *c* after the number. When a medicine has been diluted 1:10 twelve times (with vigorous shaking between each dilution), the medicine is considered a 12x. If this medicine was diluted 1:100 twelve times, it is considered a 12c.

Both of these types of potencies are effective. When recommendations for a specific potency (such as 6 or 30) are made in this book, no differentiation is made between x and c potencies because homeopaths generally do not consider the effects of these two potencies to be significantly different.

Despite using such small doses of medicines, over two hundred years of homeopathic practice has confirmed that the more a homeopathic substance has been potentized, the longer and deeper it acts and the fewer doses are needed.

After the medicines have been diluted and shaken, they are made with lactose or sucrose into pills, pellets, or globules (about the size of cake sprinkles). The number of pills to be taken per dose is always listed on the bottle or its packaging. Generally, two to eight pills are adequate. Some homeopathic medicines from the plant kingdom are made into tinctures (alcohol-based solutions), ointments, lotions, gels, or creams.

There are several important factors to keep in mind when taking homeopathic remedies to ensure their effectiveness. For best results, it is recommended that you:

- avoid touching the medicines with your hands (when taking them, pour the pills into a clean spoon or inside the bottle's cap);
- place the medicine under the tongue and let it dissolve;
- avoid eating food or drinking anything but water for fifteen minutes before or after taking a homeopathic medicine (gum, toothpaste, and cough drops should also be avoided);
- avoid drinking coffee, strong brews of herbal teas, or using camphorated products (such as cough drops, lip balm, Ben-Gay, or Tiger Balm) during the days that you are taking a homeopathic medicine (these substances can antidote the action of a remedy);
- keep the medicines in a place where there are no strong odors or bright lights.

The most economical way to purchase homeopathic medicines is to get a homeopathic medicine kit, available by mail order and through select health-food stores.

▼

For further information about homeopathy, contact the following sources (the first two are sources of books and medicine kits; all three offer general information on homeopathy):

Homeopathic Educational Services
2124 Kittredge St.
Berkeley, CA 94704
(510) 649-0294 (catalog)
(800) 359-9051 (orders)

National Center for Homeopathy
801 N. Fairfax #306
Alexandria, VA 22314
(703) 548-7790

International Foundation for Homeopathy
2366 Eastlake Dr., E.
Seattle, WA 98102
(206) 324-8230

Herbs are available at most natural-food stores in either bulk, tea bag, or capsule form. If the herbs you want are not readily available, the following companies can send herbs to you via mail order. The first three primarily sell bulk herbs, while the last (Nature's Way) primarily sells capsulated herbs.

Indiana Botanic Gardens
Box 5
Hammond, IN 46325
(219) 947-4040

Fox River Naturals
Dept. BC, Box 2
Wilmot, WI 53192
(414) 862-2395

Herb and Spice Collection
Box 118
Norway, IA 52318
(800) 365-4372

Nature's Way
10 Mountain Springs Parkway
Springville, UT 84663
(800) 926-8883

RECOMMENDED READING LIST
▼

This book hopefully whetted your appetite for learning more about natural healing. Some of the following books provide an overview of natural healing concepts, while others recommend specific strategies for healing. They will all help enhance your understanding of natural medicine and contribute to your health and happiness.

General Health Books

Achterberg, Jeanne. *Imagery in Healing.* Boston: Shambhala, 1985.

This book describes the history and present application of visualization in healing. Describing the physiological pathways that connect mind and body, the author provides sound rationale for using this healing technique. Specific visualization exercises are also included.

Carroll, David. *The Complete Book of Natural Medicines.* New York: Summit, 1980.

This book presents an overview of the principles of various natural therapies and then provides specific practical treatments for common complaints. Homeopathic medicines, herbal remedies, nutrition, and acupressure are the most commonly recommended strategies.

Castleman, Michael. *Cold Cures.* New York: Fawcett, 1987.

Covering both conventional and natural therapies, the author describes what works and what doesn't for treating colds.

Dadd, Debra Lynn. *Nontoxic, Natural, and Earthwise.* Los Angeles: Jeremy Tarcher, 1990.

The author is one of America's leading experts on the health effects of consumer products. This book is an invaluable guide to what specific products you should avoid and the natural alternatives available.

Duncan, Alice Likowski. *Your Healthy Child.* Los Angeles: Jeremy Tarcher, 1991.

This comprehensive resource guide describes natural remedies for the treatment of over one hundred common childhood ailments, emphasizing the use of nutrition, herbs, homeopathy, and acupressure. It also includes information on how a conventional physician would treat each ailment, and guidelines for when to seek professional help.

Gach, Michael Reed. *Acupressure's Potent Points.* New York: Bantam, 1990.

Written by one of the most prominent educators on acupressure, this book is a description of the most valuable and pow-

201

erful acupressure points for relieving common conditions and improving overall health.

Gardner, Joy. *The New Healing Yourself.* Freedom, CA: Crossing Press, 1989.
A mixture of new and old folk wisdom are interspersed in this practical guidebook.

Graedon, Joe. *The People's Pharmacy.* New York: St. Martins, 1985.
Written by one of the leading contemporary educators about conventional drugs, this book is an invaluable guide to learning which drugs should be avoided and which drugs are at least relatively safe.

Grist, Liz. *A Woman's Guide to Alternative Medicine.* Chicago: Contemporary, 1988.
Integrating herbal medicine, nutrition, homeopathy, bodywork, and relaxation techniques, this book provides practical advice for treating common health problems in women.

Hittleman, Richard. *Introduction to Yoga.* New York: Bantam, 1969.
One of the best introductory guides to hatha yoga, this book describes how to do the basic yogic postures. Every page includes one or more photos that help demonstrate the proper way to do each position.

Hoffman, Ronald. *Seven Weeks to a Settled Stomach.* New York: Simon and Schuster, 1990.
This comprehensive and up-to-date book describes common digestive problems and specific ways that people can prevent and treat these conditions. This is a truly impressive book that draws from the most recent medical studies and integrates conventional and alternative therapies based on them.

Israel, Richard. *The Natural Pharmacy Product Guide.* New York: Avery, 1991.
If you're confused by the overwhelming variety of natural health products available, this book is a useful consumer guide to determining the best quality brand-name products available in your health-food store. Take it with you when you wish to stock or expand your natural medicine cabinet.

Iyengar, B. K. S. *Light on Yoga.* New York: Schocken, 1979.
This five hundred plus-page book is perhaps the most complete book on hatha yoga. Written by one of the leading teachers of hatha yoga, it includes hundreds of helpful photos of the various yoga postures.

Klein, Allen. *The Healing Power of Humor.* Los Angeles: Jeremy Tarcher, 1989.
A book full of humorous stories, insights about why humor heals, and profound perceptions about what healing really is.

Locke, Stephen, and Douglas Colligan. *The Healer Within.* New York: Mentor, 1986.
This book presents an overview of the emerging field of psychoneuroimmunology, which is leading to an understanding of the physiological roadmaps that connect the mind and the body. Specific strategies of using the mind to heal the body are also described.

Ornish, Dean. *Dr. Dean Ornish's Program for Reversing Heart Disease.* New York: Random House, 1990.
Drawing from the most recent research (including the author's), this book describes a scientifically tested program for reversing heart disease. The program integrates low-fat nutrition, exercise, yoga, and stress management. A series of gourmet low-fat recipes is included.

Ornstein, Robert, and David Sobel. *Healthy Pleasures.* New York: Addison-Wesley, 1990.
Experiencing pleasure is not only fun, but can also be healing, and this book describes research that proves it. This insightful book is a pleasure to read.

Prevention editors. *The Doctor's Book of Home Remedies.* Emmaus, PA: Rodale, 1990.

Hundreds of physicians, both conventional and alternative, were asked for their favorite home remedies. This book is chockful of practical ways to heal yourself.

Schmidt, Michael. *Childhood Ear Infections.* Berkeley: North Atlantic, 1990.

Providing a comprehensive review of conventional and alternative treatments for this common pediatric affliction, the author has written a truly superb and practical book. Drawing from the medical literature, the author shows that antibiotics and ear tubes are often ineffective and tend to increase rather than decrease problems.

Standway, Andrew. *The Natural Family Doctor.* New York: Fireside, 1987.

This beautifully illustrated book is full of sound, practical information about healing common health problems.

Van Straten, Michael. *The Complete Natural Health Consultant.* New York: Prentice Hall, 1987.

An A–Z reference guide to treating common complaints, this book provides both general medical information about each condition and natural therapies to treat it.

Weil, Andrew. *Health and Healing.* Boston: Houghton Mifflin, 1983.

This book, written by the nation's leading authority on natural health care, describes the philosophical basis of both conventional and alternative medicine and is perhaps one of the best books for understanding their similarities and differences. An excellent overview book.

———. *Natural Health, Natural Medicine.* Boston: Houghton Mifflin, 1990.

This follow-up to his earlier book is a no-nonsense overview of what it takes to live a healthy life, with specific reference to how to avoid heart disease and cancer and how to protect your immune system.

Nutrition, exercise, stress management, and herbal medicine are highlighted.

Nutrition

Carper, Jean. *The Food Pharmacy.* New York: Bantam, 1988.

This well-researched and fascinating book provides folkloric and contemporary scientific information about foods and their healing powers.

Davies, Stephen, and Alan Stewart. *Nutritional Medicine.* New York: Avon, 1987.

Written by two nutrition-oriented physicians, this book provides up-to-date information about the health value of foods, vitamins, and minerals.

Gallagher, John. *Good Health with Vitamins and Minerals.* New York: Summit, 1990.

This book provides a review of vitamins and minerals, their food sources, recommended doses, risk groups for possible deficiencies, proven and unproven benefits, and toxic symptoms.

Null, Gary. *The Complete Guide to Sensible Eating.* New York: Four Walls Eight Windows, 1990.

This comprehensive sourcebook on nutrition provides up-to-date information on the nutrient content in foods and the value and potential problems of supplementation with vitamins and minerals. Specific chapters on weight management and nutrition and exercise are included, as is a detailed section that provides recipes.

Reuben, Carolyn, and Joan Priestly. *Essential Supplements for Women.* New York: Pedigree, 1989.

Written by a physician and acupuncturist/journalist, this book gives much practical advice that is drawn from clinical practice and recent research.

Robbins, John. *Diet for a New America.* Walpole, NH: Stillpoint, 1987.

This seminal book gives a comprehensive analysis of the nutritional, political, and ecological impact of food, ultimately proving with a startling array of statistics and research the significant health and environmental problems caused by our consumption of meat and dairy products.

Homeopathic Medicines

Cummings, Stephen, and Dana Ullman. *Everybody's Guide to Homeopathic Medicines, Revised and Expanded.* Los Angeles: Jeremy Tarcher, 1991.

This practical guidebook to using homeopathic medicines provides the rationale for using these remedies for common health problems and gives indications for when professional care is recommended.

Panos, Maesimund, and Jane Heimlich. *Homeopathic Medicine at Home.* Los Angeles: Jeremy Tarcher, 1980.

Though not as comprehensive as *Everybody's Guide to Homeopathic Medicines*, this book provides helpful charts that aid the finding of the correct homeopathic remedy.

Ullman, Dana. *Discovering Homeopathy: Medicine for the 21st Century.* Berkeley: North Atlantic, 1991.

For skeptic and advocate alike, this book is a solid introduction to homeopathic medicine. Various contemporary health problems are discussed in the light of this valuable approach to healing.

Herbs

Castleman, Michael. *The Healing Herbs.* Emmaus, PA: Rodale, 1991.

Integrating modern scientific information with folklore, the author has written an immensely valuable book that is both practical and intellectually stimulating.

Tierra, Michael. *The Way of Herbs.* New York: Pocket, 1990.

This popular herbal guide teaches you how to use 130 Western herbs and 40 Chinese herbs. The author teaches you how to make the various kinds of herbal preparations. He also gives his own special formulas for specific ailments.

Theiss, Barbara and Peter. *The Family Herbal.* Rochester, VT: Healing Arts, 1989.

Drawing from the European herbal tradition, the authors describe numerous applications for forty herbs. Beautiful photos of the herbs and how to apply them are interspersed throughout the book.

Magazines, Newsletters, and Journals

Natural Health, formerly *East West Journal,* 17 Station St., Box 1200, Brookline, MA 02147.

Perhaps the most sophisticated monthly health magazine in the U.S., *East West* focuses on health issues and controversies, usually with an ecological perspective and an integration of Eastern and Western thought.

The Edell Health Letter, 475 Gate Five Rd., Sausalito, CA 94965.

This eight-page monthly newsletter provides short blurbs of provocative and practical health information drawn from medical journals.

Health Facts, 237 Thompson St., New York, NY 10012.

With its roots in consumer rights and patient advocacy, this eight-page monthly newsletter provides solid information and helpful resources.

HerbalGram, P.O. Box 201660, Austin, TX 78720.

No other magazine offers this level of sophisticated information on the use of herbs as medicines. A quarterly magazine.

Longevity, 1965 Broadway, New York, NY 10023-5965.

This monthly magazine not only includes articles on how to prolong life but also on how to improve the quality of the life you live. It provides a good balance between the cutting edge of medical science and that of the healing arts.

Medical Abstracts Newsletter, P.O. Box 2170, Teaneck, NJ 07666.

This six-page monthly newsletter provides abstracts of clinical research in general medicine, pediatrics, heart disease, cancer, obstetrics and gynecology, sexual medicine, psychiatry, aging, and sports medicine. It is invaluable in helping to keep up with new research.

New Age Journal, 342 Western, Brighton, MA 02146.

Although this isn't primarily a health magazine, it does regularly publish thoughtful and practical health articles on the leading edge of current awareness. Bimonthly.

People's Medical Society Newsletter, 462 Walnut St., Allentown, PA 18102.

This eight-page monthly newsletter informs consumers how to use their doctor and hospital effectively and economically. Its articles commonly warn people of medical procedures or drugs that have been found to be ineffective or dangerous. Al-though few articles actually describe alternatives to conventional medicine, this important newsletter provides you with good reasons to seek them.

The Townsend Letter for Doctors, 911 Tyler St., Port Townsend, WA 98368.

A truly rich resource, this one hundred-page monthly magazine is primarily directed at doctors who are practicing alternative medicine, though anyone can benefit from reading it. In addition to numerous articles, each issue has many abstracts of research, book reviews, and discussions of legal and political issues in health care.

The U.C. Berkeley Wellness Letter, P.O. Box 420148, Palm Coast, FL 32142.

Drawing from the latest conventional medical literature, this eight-page monthly newsletter provides reliable health information that people can readily use.

Yoga Journal, 2054 University Ave., Berkeley, CA 94704.

Despite its name, this monthly magazine does not just discuss yoga. Each issue also contains articles on health issues, spiritual practice, relaxation strategies, and consciousness studies.

ABOUT THE AUTHOR

▼

Dana Ullman, M.P.H. received his masters degree in public health from the University of California at Berkeley, specializing in health education.

He has written two books, *Everybody's Guide to Homeopathic Medicines* and *Discovering Homeopathy: Medicine for the 21st Century*, and is presently completing a book on treating infants and children with homeopathic medicines. He is also the health-book reviewer for the *Utne Reader*.

Ullman founded the Foundation for Homeopathic Education and Research, in collaboration with professors at Harvard, Yale, University of California at San Francisco, U.C.L.A., and several other medical schools. He also serves on the Board of Directors of the National Center for Homeopathy and has organized their annual conferences since 1986.

His company, Homeopathic Educational Services in Berkeley, is the country's largest publisher and distributor of homeopathic books, tapes, medicines, medicine kits, software, and general information.

He has not, however, simply been interested in specific healing practices but also in the public policy implications of these methods. To this end, he organized conferences for or served as a consultant to University of California at Berkeley, the federal Department of Health and Human Services, the California Medical Board, and The San Francisco Foundation.

He is married and lives in Oakland, California.

FEEDBACK

I am interested in hearing about your experiences with this book's one-minute strategies. I am also interested in knowing if you have your own effective one-minute strategies to share. Please write to me at the address below with your input.

Dana Ullman
2124 Kittredge St.
Berkeley, CA 94704